Headache and Facial Pain

T0177886

What Do I Do Now?

SERIES CO-EDITORS-IN-CHIEF

Lawrence C. Newman, MD
Director, Headache Division NYU Langone Health
Professor of Neurology
NYU Grossman School of Medicine
New York, New York

Morris Levin, MD
Director of the Headache Center
Professor of Neurology
University of California, San Francisco
San Francisco, California

OTHER VOLUMES IN THE SERIES

Headache and Facial Pain

SECOND EDITION

Lawrence C. Newman, MD
Director, Headache Division NYU Langone Health
Professor of Neurology, NYU Grossman School of Medicine
New York, NY

Morris Levin, MD
Professor, Department of Neurology
University of California, San Francisco
San Francisco, CA

Rashmi B. Halker Singh, MD, FAHS, FAAN
Associate Professor of Neurology
Director, Headache Medicine Fellowship Program
Division of Headache Medicine
Department of Neurology
Mayo Clinic
Scottsdale, AZ

Rebecca L. Michael, MD
Assistant Clinical Professor
Division of Headache and Facial Pain
Department of Neurology
University of California, San Francisco
San Francisco, CA

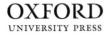

OXFORD
UNIVERSITY PRESS

OXFORD
UNIVERSITY PRESS

Oxford University Press is a department of the University of Oxford. It furthers
the University's objective of excellence in research, scholarship, and education
by publishing worldwide. Oxford is a registered trade mark of Oxford University
Press in the UK and certain other countries.

Published in the United States of America by Oxford University Press
198 Madison Avenue, New York, NY 10016, United States of America.

© Oxford University Press 2022

Library of Congress Cataloging-in-Publication Data
Names: Newman, Lawrence C., M.D., author. | Levin, Morris, 1955– author. |
Halker Singh, Rashmi B., author. | Michael, Rebecca L., author.
Title: Headache and facial pain / Lawrence C. Newman, Morris Levin,
Rashmi B. Halker Singh, Rebecca L. Michael.
Other titles: What do I do now?
Description: 2. | New York, NY : Oxford University Press, [2022]. |
Series: What do I do now? | Includes bibliographical references and index.
Identifiers: LCCN 2021046072 (print) | LCCN 2021046073 (ebook) |
ISBN 9780190842130 (paperback) | ISBN 9780190842154 (epub) |
ISBN 9780190842161
Subjects: MESH: Headache—diagnosis | Headache—therapy | Headache
Disorders—diagnosis | Headache Disorders—therapy | Facial Pain—diagnosis |
Facial Pain—therapy | Diagnosis, Differential | Case Reports
Classification: LCC RC392 (print) | LCC RC392 (ebook) | NLM WL 342 |
DDC 616.8/491—dc23
LC record available at https://lccn.loc.gov/2021046072
LC ebook record available at https://lccn.loc.gov/2021046073

DOI: 10.1093/med/9780190842130.001.0001

9 8 7 6 5 4 3 2 1

Printed by Marquis, Canada

Dr. Lawrence Newman

To Dad.

Dr. Morris Levin

To my wife Karen—for your love, support, and creative criticism; to my father Hy—for your model of purpose and perseverance; to my mother Leah—for your enthusiasm and encouragement; to my mentors, colleagues, and students; and to my patients.

Dr. Rashmi Halker Singh

To Neil—the person I always inevitably turn to when I need advice regarding "What do I do now?" with life's various challenges. And to Mira—as a general life lesson, if the "What do I do now?" question involves a travel opportunity or a rescue dog, the correct answer is probably yes.

Dr. Rebecca L. Michael

To my father, who has always been an inspiration and mentor for me throughout my journey as a physician.

Contents

Diagnostic Questions

1 Orgasmic Headaches

A 28-year-old man with a history of occasional "stress" headaches describes a new type of headache occurring intermittently during the past several weeks. It is severe ("blinding"), bifrontal, and occurs abruptly only at or near the time of orgasm. There have been approximately six to eight of these. They do not always occur with intercourse—"about every third or fourth time." These do not occur with any other activity and have been so severe as to induce him to at times abstain from sex. He has been tried unsuccessfully on beta-blocker prophylaxis. Computed tomography (CT) of the head and CT angiography (CTA) have been normal. His wife is scared that "he has an aneurysm" that was missed on imaging because his father "died from one." The headaches have led to marital discord.

What do you do now?

A severe abrupt headache occurring with exertion is suggestive of sub-arachnoid hemorrhage (SAH), other intracranial hemorrhage, or arterial dissection. Thus, it must be aggressively worked up. Recurring exertional or sex-induced headaches, as in this case, paint a different, more benign picture—usually. Nevertheless, it is imperative to rule out serious causes of sudden or "thunderclap headache" (Box 1.1), including ruptured berry aneurysm, intracranial hemorrhage, cervical arterial dissection, and cerebral venous thrombosis (CVT).

Aneurysmal SAH may present without neurological signs initially, so CT of the head and lumbar puncture are essential. If some time has passed, diagnosis is, of course, more challenging. Intracranial hemorrhage, particularly if small, may also present rather benignly, but neuroimaging is generally unambiguous. CVT may be missed without a magnetic resonance (MR) or CT venogram. Assessment by MR angiography (MRA) of the carotids and vertebral arteries should exclude cervical arterial dissection. Another entity that can present rather deceptively is reversible cerebral vasoconstriction

---

BOX 1.1 **Causes of Sudden (Thunderclap) Headache**

Subarachnoid hemorrhage or "aneurismal leak" (sentinel headache)
Intraparenchymal hemorrhage, lobar, or pituitary intracranial
  hemorrhage
Cerebral venous thrombosis
Carotid or vertebral artery dissection
Intracranial hypotension
Cerebral vasculitis (primary or systemic)
Reversible cerebral vasoconstriction syndrome
Acute hypertension
Sphenoid sinusitis
Meningitis
Acute paranasal sinusitis
Primary thunderclap headache
Primary exercise headache
Sex-related headache
Cardiac cephalalgia

syndrome (RCVS), previously known as "Call–Fleming syndrome." This generally presents with sudden or severe headaches, sometimes in a series over days to weeks, and later possibly with neurological deficits due to ischemic brain injury. Unlike central nervous system vasculitis, cerebrospinal fluid in RCVS is generally normal, and brain MR imaging (MRI) is often normal as well. The hallmark is the finding of segmental arterial narrowing seen on angiography, similar to that seen in arteritis. Noncontrast brain CT often reveals small focal SAHs, presumably the cause of previous thunderclap headaches. Meningitis and acute bacterial sinusitis are not generally missed because their accompanying features, such as fever, meningismus, and sinus tenderness, are so suggestive. Intracranial hypotension may cause sudden severe headaches for unclear reasons (see Chapter 8). These patients often, but not always, provide a history of significant worsening of pain when arising. Significant hypertension, as is seen in pheochromocytoma or uncontrolled idiopathic hypertension, is easily discovered. Occasionally, intracranial brain neoplasms can present with thunderclap headache, as can hydrocephalus. Finally, the rare entity of third ventricle colloid cyst can produce a sudden headache due to the ball-valve nature of its anatomy leading to rapid increases in intracranial pressure.

The differential diagnosis in sex-related headaches also includes primary exertional headaches and primary thunderclap headaches (see Chapter 14). These may last for a number of hours and are also of rapid onset. Whether benign exertional headaches, primary thunderclap headaches, and sex-related headaches represent different manifestations of the same underlying condition remains to be determined. There is one other potential diagnosis to consider in sex-related headaches—cardiac cephalalgia. This rare phenomenon involves significant headache at the time of cardiac ischemia, the mechanism of which must relate to some unknown pain referral pattern. It is diagnosed cardiologically and, in a way, can be a fortunate warning sign for treatable coronary ischemia (Table 1.1).

So, how aggressively must the workup be here? Given the recurring, virtually pathognomonic, nature of these headaches, it is tempting to fit them neatly into the category of the orgasmic headache (also known as primary headache associated with sexual activity), classically defined as sudden severe headaches occurring near or at the time of orgasm. A brain MRI to rule out recent hemorrhage, MRA or CTA of the cerebral vessels to investigate

TABLE 1.1 Exertional and Sexual Headaches

Type	Characteristics
Primary cough headache	Bilateral severe short headaches brought on by any Valsalva maneuvers (important to exclude skull base lesion including Chiari malformation)
Primary exercise headache	Unilateral or bilateral, emerges during exercise, usually in young males, lasting up to 48 hours
Orgasmic headache	Severe explosive, frontal or occipital, occurring at the time of orgasm lasting up to 72 hours
Positional sexual headache	Suboccipital, following intercourse, worse with upright position (thought to be due to dural cerebrospinal fluid leak), lasting days without treatment
Cardiac cephalalgia	Severe headache during cardiac ischemia, may be unaccompanied by angina, diagnosed with electrocardiogram and cardiac evaluation

for aneurysm and segmental narrowing, MRA of the cervical vessels to look for dissection, and MR venography to rule out CVT would be a very thorough approach. But is this even enough? When a family member has (or had) a known intracranial berry aneurysm(s), the chance of an aneurysm in an individual may be as much as four times greater than the average risk (general prevalence of cerebral aneurysms is 1–5%). When patients and families remain concerned, conventional angiography can give a definitive answer, but risks must be weighed.

A parsimonious diagnostic scenario in this case might be as follows:

1. Thorough medical and neurological examination reveals no deficits, including fundoscopy.
2. MRI of the brain reveals no abnormalities.
3. Treatment leads to adequate resolution of the headaches.

Later, questions of further screening for aneurysm can be discussed, and close observation for new clues can continue.

Treatment options are reasonably good for orgasmic headache. Indomethacin 25–50 mg approximately 1 hour prior to intercourse is often successful at completely preventing an attack. Beta-blockers such as propranolol, atenolol, or metoprolol can be effective in case prophylaxis makes more sense (frequency, convenience). A relative contraindication is the possibility of impotence due to these drugs, which can further worsen the marital problem already surfacing. Calcium channel blockers have also been tried. Altering sexual positions has been reported to help. Acutely, triptans have been effective, and nonsteroidal anti-inflammatory medications in addition to indomethacin have been useful for many patients as well.

KEY POINTS TO REMEMBER

· Exertional and sexual headaches are benign primary headaches, but their presentations may indicate underlying structural disease.

· Thunderclap headache—a sudden severe headache of any type—may also indicate underlying vascular or other organic pathology, including cerebral aneurysm, CVT, arterial dissection, and RCVS.

· When a family member has a known berry aneurysm(s), the chance of an aneurysm in an individual may be as much as four times greater than the average risk.

· As is true for several other primary headache disorders, primary orgasmic headache seems to be particularly responsive to indomethacin.

Further Reading

Ari BC, Domac FM, Ulutas S. Primary headache associated with sexual activity: A case series of 13 patients. *J Clin Neurosci*. 2020;79:51–53.

Bahra A. Other primary headaches—Thunderclap-, cough-, exertional-, and sexual headache. *J Neurol*. 2020;4:1–3.

Frese A, Eikermann A, Frese K, et al. Headache associated with sexual activity: Demography, clinical features, and comorbidity. *Neurology*. 2003;61:796–800.

Ronkainen A, Miettinen H, Karkola K, et al. Risk of harboring an unruptured intracranial aneurysm. *Stroke*. 1998;29:359–362.

2 Sinus Headache

A 45-year-old park ranger has had frequent severe
"sinus" headaches for several years. There is often
nasal discharge. They are generally bifrontal or
centered over the bridge of his nose. They are often
worsened by bending forward. He develops mild
nausea with the most severe ones, as well as some
degree of photophobia. Antibiotic courses have
helped on occasion, but headaches tend to return
once the treatment ends. Sumatriptan and rizatriptan
have been of some use, but he is frequently using
over-the-counter (OTC) medications on most days for
pain. His medical exam is normal with no particular
intensification of pain with palpation over the frontal,
maxillary, or ethmoid sinuses. Magnetic resonance
imaging (MRI) of the head reveals maxillary and
sphenoid sinus hyperdensities (Figure 2.1).

What do you do now?

ere, diagnosis is a bit complicated. There are plenty of migraine features (Box 2.1)—for example, nausea, photophobia, and chronicity—but there are also some features suggestive of a nasal or paranasal sinus pain origin—nasal discharge, worsening with dependent position, response to antibiotics (albeit temporarily), and the MRI findings. Because it is well known that triptans may abort nonmigrainous headaches of many types (including even the headache of subarachnoid hemorrhage), the response to triptans is not diagnostic either.

The *International Classification of Headache Disorders*, third edition, requires that diagnosis of "Headaches attributed to rhinosinusitis" be supported by imaging and examination evidence, which this patient does seem to have. His headache also seems to remit after sinusitis treatment, another requirement (Box 2.2). But why do headaches keep returning? And could the daily use of OTC medications be exacerbating an underlying migraine physiology via the mechanism of medication overuse headache?

The confounding issue, of course, is the high prevalence of primary headache disorders as well as sinus-type symptoms in the general population. Many patients self-diagnose "sinus headaches," which leads to much overuse of sinus remedies. This can in turn lead to a rebounding of sinus-type symptoms—particularly increasingly more sinus congestion. When these approaches seem to be failing, clinicians can become more liberal with antibiotic prescriptions, which may or may not lessen the headaches.

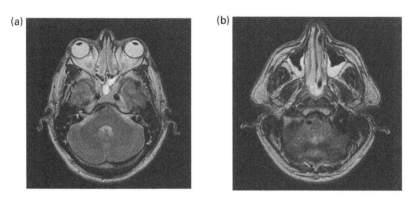

(a)　　　　　　　　(b)

FIGURE 2.1 Sphenoid sinus (a) and bilateral maxillary sinus (b) hyperdensities. (Courtesy of John J. McIntyre, MD, Section of Neuroradiology, Dartmouth Hitchcock Medical Center, Lebanon, NH.)

Paranasal sinus imaging has become accurate enough to rule out cases of sinusitis that require surgical and/or medical treatment. When imaging of the nasal and paranasal regions is negative, most clinicians will move on to other lines of investigation, although the possibility of nonvisualizable chronic sinus pathology persists. When sinus imaging is positive, things are not so straightforward. Does a maxillary polyp hold significance in patients with primarily headache? Probably not. What about "mucosal changes"? Again—probably not important. Key imaging findings that suggest significant sinus pathology include (1) tissue changes filling one or more sinus cavities; (2) air–fluid levels in maxillary, ethmoid, frontal, or sphenoid sinuses; and (3) evidence of bony or other tissue deformity. Of interest is a study by Hansen et al. (the HUNT study) showing a distinct lack of correlation between paranasal sinus opacification on imaging and headaches. The best approach in some of these cases, particularly those unresponsive to antibiotics, is to enlist the aid of a skilled otolaryngologist. Endoscopic evaluation and biopsy of sinus tissue is possible, and fungal, parasitic, or resistant/unusual bacterial infections have been discovered in this way.

In the previous case, it is crucial to try noninvasive measures aimed at migraine, medication overuse headache, and improving sinus hygiene. The sphenoid sinus opacification is of concern but not crucially so, particularly if repeat imaging shows no progression of imaging changes. Prophylactic medication for migraine such as beta-blocker, cyclic antidepressant, anticonvulsant, or calcitonin gene-related peptide modulating treatment should be considered. Discontinuation of all unnecessary OTC medication should certainly be done. In this case, nasal/sinus irrigation and a thorough search for allergic triggers should be undertaken if not already done. If these measures fail, endoscopic evaluation seems sensible, including biopsy, in the hope of finding a treatable cause for the sinus-related component of the patient's headaches.

On a more controversial plane, there are in fact a number of otolaryngological conditions that are thought by some to cause headache. These include (1) concha bullosa (an expanded turbinate with an internal air cell), (2) nasal septal deviation, (3) septal spurs (sharp bony projections off the septum that can impinge on lateral nasal wall tissues), and (4) rhinolithiasis (foreign bodies trapped in the nasal cavity). The close impingement of mucosal sinus tissues ("contact points") caused by these processes may cause stimulation of nasal branches of the maxillary nerve, leading to local and referred head pain.

KEY POINTS TO REMEMBER

- When patients present with "sinus headaches" as well as some migraine features, it is always best to follow the trails of both, with workup and treatment aimed at discovering all relevant diagnoses.

- Imaging findings suggestive of sinus-related headaches include filling opacity in one or more sinus cavities; air–fluid levels in maxillary, ethmoid, frontal, or sphenoid sinuses; and evidence of bony changes involving the surrounding osseous structures.
- Endoscopic evaluation, including biopsy, can be diagnostic if noninvasive measures fail.

Further Reading

Cady RK, Schreiber CP. Sinus headache or migraine? Considerations in making a differential diagnosis. *Neurology*. 2002;58:S10–S14.

Eross, E, Dodick, DW, Eross, M. The Sinus, Allergy and Migraine Study (SAMS). *Headache*. 2007;47:213–224.

Hansen AG, Stovner LJ, Hagen K, Helvik AS, et al. Paranasal sinus opacification in headache sufferers: A population-based imaging study (the HUNT study–MRI). *Cephalalgia*. 2017;37:509–516.

Headache Classification Committee of the International Headache Society. The *International Classification of Headache Disorders*, 3rd edition. *Cephalalgia*. 2018;38:1–211.

Rank MA, Hoxworth JM, Lal D. Sorting out "sinus headache." *J Allergy Clin Immunol: In Practice*. 2016;4:1013–1014.

3 White Matter Abnormalities on Magnetic Resonance Imaging

Specialties: Neurology, Radiology, and Primary Care

A 46-year-old woman presents with a 20-year history of bilateral, throbbing headaches with associated nausea, rare vomiting, and sensitivity to lights, sounds, and smells. Until the past 6 months, her headaches were under good control, occurring approximately two or three times per month and sometimes with her menstrual cycle. She would treat them with either ibuprofen or naproxen and would experience relief within 2 or 3 hours. In the past 6 months, these headaches have become more frequent, and are now occurring at least once a week, and nonsteroidal anti-inflammatory drugs (NSAIDs) are not consistently helpful. Her paternal aunt has a history of brain tumor, and she is worried about her increase in headache frequency. When asked about any aura symptoms, she reports right arm numbness accompanying some of her headaches. The patient's medical and neurological examinations are normal. Because of her headache pattern change and the focal arm symptoms, you order magnetic resonance imaging (MRI) of the brain, which reveals scattered white matter hyperintensities (WMH) on T2 (Figure 3.1). The radiologist's report states that demyelinating disease must be excluded.

What do you do now?

White matter hyperintensities are a common incidental finding on brain MRI, occurring in approximately 10% of people aged 30–40 years. The prevalence of WMH increases with age, and they are also seen more commonly in individuals with hypertension, diabetes, hypercholesterolemia, cerebrovascular and cardiovascular disease, multiple sclerosis (MS), and collagen vascular and other autoimmune disorders. Because the causes of WMH are so extensive, determining their etiology can at times be difficult.

Although most people with migraine have normal MRIs, the most common MRI abnormality seen is WMH. The prevalence of WMH in migraine ranges from 12% to 46%. These abnormalities are usually characterized by small, multiple, punctate hyperintensities that are best seen on both T2-weighted and fluid attenuation inversion recovery (FLAIR) sequences. The WMH of migraine are typically bilateral and most often located in the deep white matter, but the localization in migraine varies with age. Prior to age 40 years, people with migraine are more likely to have these WMH in the centrum semiovale and frontal subcortical white matter. After age 40 years, the lesions are predominantly localized in the deeper white matter, at the level of the basal ganglia.

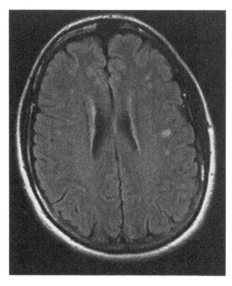

FIGURE 3.1 Typical white matter lesions of migraine on magnetic resonance imaging.

People with migraine are four times more likely than people without migraine to have WMH on MRI. This increased risk is independent of age and vascular risk factors. Although there does not appear to be an association between the presence or severity of periventricular WMH and migraine, there is a twofold risk for lesions in the deep white matter in women with migraine. This risk is highest in women who experience more than one migraine monthly.

The cause of WMH in migraine is not known. In general, hyperintensities in these areas are thought to be the result of ischemic damage or demyelination, so either of these processes may occur in migraine. It has been postulated that WMH that occur in migraine may be secondary to abnormal platelet aggregation with subsequent microemboli, hypoperfusion states that occur during aura, or cerebrovascular dysregulation. Perhaps focal hypermetabolic phenomena occur during migraine, leading to an "outstripping" of the blood supply, resulting in focal ischemic injuries.

Among the myriad causes of WMH, those that occur with headaches as a significant manifestation include migraine with and without aura, mitochondrial encephalopathy with lactic acidosis and stroke-like episodes (MELAS), cerebral autosomal dominant arteriopathy with subcortical infarcts and leukoencephalopathy (CADASIL), central nervous system vasculitis, systemic vasculitides that involve cerebral arteries, anticardiolipin antibody syndrome, and MS. The WMH in these disorders differ in their location, appearance, and numbers. The WMH of CADASIL are symmetrical and confluent and are best visualized on T2 and FLAIR sequences. These WMH are most prominent in the frontal and anterior temporal lobes and are associated with diffuse lacunar-type infarcts in the deep white matter and basal ganglia. The MRI changes in MELAS have a predilection for the occipital and temporal lobes and involve both gray and white matter. The MRI lesions in vasculitis also affect the gray and white matter, and the WMH tend to be contrast-enhancing. The hyperintensities in MS resemble those seen in migraine but, unlike migraine, involve the corpus callosum, cerebellum, and brainstem. The appearance of the periventricular WMH in MS differs as well. Rather than the small, punctate findings of migraine, MS produces ovoid lesions that align perpendicularly to the ventricles ("Dawson's fingers").

The absence of a family history of recurrent strokes and dementia and only one family member with migraine make CADASIL unlikely in this patient. Similarly, MELAS can be eliminated by the clinical history. A prior history of fetal loss, thrombosis, and thrombocytopenia would be expected in the anticardiolipin syndrome and is not reported by this patient. Many patients with MS report migraine-like headaches, and it is important to clarify for current or previous symptoms that might be suggestive of MS, as well as carefully evaluate the distribution and location of lesions on MRI. The new onset of numbness in this woman together with the abnormalities on her MRI make this a possibility. Indeed, in the early stages of MS, the WMH are quite similar to those seen in migraine (and in this patient). However, the location of the WMH in this case is much more typical for migraine than for MS. Specifically, the MRI demonstrates scattered punctate lesions in the centrum semiovale and frontal regions.

No further investigations are needed for our patient at this time. Her history and MRI findings are characteristic of migraine, and the numbness is almost certainly a sensory aura. However, should her complaints change, or her neurological examination become abnormal, she should be reevaluated, and additional testing can be done. At that point, repeat MRI can assess for change in lesion count and location. Lumbar puncture might be appropriate for evaluation of possible demyelinating or inflammatory disease. Evoked potentials can be done to assess for subclinical demyelinating disease.

The other question that often arises is one of management. If these WMH in fact represent some form of ischemic damage, might prophylaxis with aspirin or another platelet antiaggregant medication be reasonable? At least, more careful attention might be devoted to nonpharmaceutical prophylaxis of cerebrovascular disease, such as control of blood pressure and lipid levels. There is no evidence yet to support this, but ongoing research is aimed at finding some answers.

For this patient, we can reassure her that her clinical picture is consistent with a diagnosis of migraine with and without aura. We do not need to follow her WMH with serial MRIs, and she does not need further imaging unless she develops new symptoms. The fact that her migraine attacks are becoming more frequent is concerning, and she would benefit from a prescription acute medication, such as a triptan, and also potentially being started on a preventive treatment to reduce headache frequency. Careful discussion to evaluate for potential modifiable reasons for migraine worsening is also important, and we can make sure to review her sleep patterns, external stressors, caffeine intake, acute mediation use with her NSAIDs, and also her hormonal status because perimenopause is a time when women can experience an increase in headache frequency. If any of these factors might be playing a role, addressing them will be important as well.

KEY POINTS TO REMEMBER

- White matter hyperintensities are four times more likely in individuals with migraine, particularly in women.
- White matter hyperintensities are generally small, punctate lesions, affecting deep white matter and best seen on T2 and FLAIR sequences.
- White matter hyperintensities are more common in frontal subcortical regions and the centrum semiovale before age 40 years and in deeper white matter and the basal ganglia after age 40 years.
- If there are no red flags in the history or examination, and the diagnosis is consistent with migraine, no further workup is needed for WMH.

Further Reading

Arkink EB, Palm-Meinders IH, Koppen H, et al. Microstructural white matter changes preceding white matter hyperintensities in migraine. *Neurology*. 2019;93:e688–e694.

Ashina S, Bentivegna E, Martelletti P, Eikermann-Haerter K. Structural and functional brain changes in migraine. *Pain Ther*. 2021; 10:211–223.

Kruit MC, van Buchem MA, Hofman PA, et al. Migraine as a risk factor for subclinical brain lesions. *JAMA*. 2004;291:427–434.

Palm-Meinders IH, Koppen H, Terwindt GM, et al. Structural brain changes in migraine. *JAMA*. 2012;308:1889–1897.

Porter A, Gladstone JP, Dodick DW. Migraine and white matter hyperintensities. *Curr Headache Rep*. 2005;4:141–145.

4 Giant Cell Arteritis

An 84 year-old woman complains of 3 weeks of severe right-sided headaches and shoulder pain. She reports body aches, fatigue, and pain on combing her hair. Her exam reveals a hardened right temporal artery with diminished pulsations. Her sedimentation rate is 120 mm/hour, and her C-reactive protein is 4.2 mg/dL. She takes alendronate for severe osteoporosis discovered after a hip fracture 2 years ago. Her internist is concerned about the long-term consequences of treatment with steroids.

What do you do now?

With this case, the clinician faces a dilemma. Failure to treat a patient with giant cell arteritis (GCA) portends devastating consequences, yet so too does needlessly exposing someone with advanced osteoporosis to the effects of long-term steroid use. The most common primary vasculitis in adulthood, GCA affects medium and large arteries. This inflammatory arteritis has its onset almost always after age 50 years, and the highest incidence occurs in the seventh and eighth decades of life. It affects women three times more often than men and occurs more commonly in whites than other races.

Clinically, GCA may present in a variety of ways. A new onset of headache is reported in up to 75% of patients with GCA. These headaches may be associated with constitutional symptoms such as fever, joint and muscle pains, anorexia, weight loss, and fatigue. As many as 40% of patients with GCA also have polymyalgia rheumatica. Additional findings include abnormalities of the temporal artery (beading, prominence, tenderness, and pulselessness), jaw claudication, scalp tenderness, tongue or scalp necrosis, diplopia, elevated erythrocyte sedimentation rate (ESR), and visual changes. Indeed, it is the potential for GCA to cause a rapidly sequential, bilateral blindness that makes early recognition and treatment of paramount importance. Vagaries in presentation make this disorder challenging. Although headache is reported by most patients with GCA, it is also common in many other conditions. Jaw claudication, commonly attributed to GCA, is in fact present in only 34% of sufferers. Twenty percent of patients with GCA report no systemic symptoms.

Because GCA can present with several different clinical scenarios and because many of the features of GCA are vague and nonspecific, the ability of the clinician to correctly diagnose the syndrome with a high level of sensitivity is a key concern. The American College of Rheumatology diagnostic criteria for GCA are listed in Box 4.1. The presence of three or more of these criteria yields a sensitivity of 93.5% and a specificity of 91.2%. Rodriguez-Valverde and coworkers (1997) developed an alternate set of criteria that combines clinical features and laboratory testing. In these criteria, an age of onset ≥70 years, new-onset headache, and abnormal temporal artery examination have a positive predictive value of 93%. If jaw claudication occurs in addition to the previous three criteria, the positive predictive value increases to 100%. Other positive clinical predictors, culled from a meta-analysis of patients with GCA, include, in descending order of likeliness, beading of the temporal artery, prominent or enlarged temporal artery, jaw claudication, diplopia, absent temporal artery pulse, tender temporal artery, or any temporal artery finding.

If GCA is considered likely by clinical history and physical examination, a workup demonstrating elevations in ESR and C-reactive protein (CRP) should be done. Abnormalities on these tests signal the presence of a systemic inflammatory process and should be corroborated by temporal artery biopsy (TAB). Several clinical factors predict the likelihood of a positive TAB. The likelihood ratio is a direct estimate of how much a test result will change the odds of having a disease. This ratio may be expressed as either a positive or a negative value. The likelihood ratio for a positive result tells you how much the odds of the disease increase when a test is positive. The likelihood ratio for a negative result tells you how much the odds of the disease decrease when a test is negative. The likelihood ratio of a positive TAB in patients with an abnormal ESR is 1.1. As the ESR rises above 50 mm/hour, the likelihood ratio also rises, to 1.2; and when the ESR is >100, the likelihood of a positive biopsy is 1.9. Because the ESR may be normal in approximately 17% of patients with GCA, a more useful marker is the CRP level. Elevated CRP was found in 100% of patients with biopsy-proven GCA. The sensitivity of an elevated CRP was reported to be 97.5%, and when both ESR and CRP were elevated, the sensitivity increased to 99%.

BOX 4.1 **American College of Rheumatology Criteria for Giant Cell Arteritis**

1. Age at onset ≥50 years
2. New-onset or new type of headache
3. Temporal artery tenderness to palpation or decreased pulsation, unrelated to cervical artery arteriosclerosis
4. Erythrocyte sedimentation rate ≥50 mm/hour by Westergren method
5. Abnormal temporal artery biopsy showing vasculitis characterized by a predominance of mononuclear cell infiltration or granulomatous infiltration, usually with multinucleated giant cells

Source: Melson et al. (2007).

If clinical suspicion is high, even in the presence of normal inflammatory markers, TAB should be performed because missing the diagnosis of GCA is associated with significant morbidity, whereas the risk of TAB is quite low.

Temporal artery biopsy is considered the gold standard for the diagnosis of GCA, and the yield of a positive biopsy may be optimized by taking a long sample (2–5 cm) from the symptomatic side and instructing the pathologist to examine multiple, thin, serial cuts done at small intervals. This ensures that false-negative results are minimized because GCA may cause "skip" lesions, in which segments of the vessel are affected in a discontinuous pattern. The sensitivity of a unilateral TAB is approximately 90% and is slightly higher for bilateral sections. In general, unilateral TAB is usually sufficient; however, contralateral biopsies may be performed when the first biopsy is normal in a patient in whom there is a high clinical suspicion for GCA. Although the yield of the additional biopsy is seemingly low, averaging approximately 5%, it may uncover the disease in patients with a previously false-negative biopsy.

Our patient meets the American College of Rheumatology criteria for GCA, fulfilling four of the five requirements. Furthermore, using the clinical predictors of GCA established by Smetana and Shmerling (2002), the presence of right temporal artery hardening increased the likelihood that our patient has GCA (positive likelihood ratio of 2), as does her increased ESR >100 (positive likelihood ratio of 1.9). Using the alternative diagnostic criteria of Rodriguez-Valverde et al. (1997), this patient's clinical history gives us a positive predictive value for GCA of 93%.

The overwhelming odds are that this patient does in fact have GCA, and a very good case can be made for initiating therapy with prednisone 40–60 mg daily pending the results of her TAB. The biopsy must be performed within 1 week of initiating steroid therapy to prevent a false-negative result.

Corticosteroids are considered the preferred treatment of GCA. Response to treatment is rapid; systemic features of the illness usually remit within days, and the ESR normalizes within the first week. Various treatment strategies have been described, although none have been tested in a randomized controlled study. In general, high doses are prescribed initially, maintained until symptoms resolve, and then slowly tapered with weekly monitoring of CRP and close follow-up looking for recurrence of symptoms. There is no absolute consensus on the duration of treatment, and many patients require low-dose maintenance for 2 years or more. However, in light of the potential serious consequences associated with long-term steroid use, especially in our patient who has significant osteoporosis, are there alternatives available to minimize her exposure to steroid therapy?

Tocilizumab (TCZ), an interleukin (IL)-6 receptor blocker, was approved for the treatment of GCA in 2017. When subcutaneous TCZ was added to standardized prednisone therapy, patients had faster and longer-lasting remissions and lower prednisone requirements than those receiving placebo (Stone et al. 2016). The treatment is not without risk, however. TCZ has a black box warning for serious infections.

Other steroid-sparing agents (methotrexate, cyclophosphamide, azothiaprine, and dapsone) have been tried in the treatment of GCA with suboptimal or inconsistent results. Likewise, anecdotal benefit with tumor necrosis factor inhibitors (etanercept and infliximab) has been reported. Results from randomized trials were less impressive.

For our patient, treatment should be initiated with oral prednisone 40–60 mg/day together with subcutaneous injections of TCZ 162 mg weekly. In addition to following the patient's clinical symptoms, CRP levels, liver function tests, and monitoring for neutropenia and thrombocytopenia should be done weekly. Serum glucose levels must be closely monitored and treated.

When treating CGA with systemic glucocorticoids, disease response can be measured by symptom resolution and normalization of the CRP and ESR. It is important to note that blockade of IL-6 invariably causes normalization of CRP and ESR levels via induction of hepatic synthesis of acute phase reactants. Therefore, in patients treated with TCZ, the clinician must closely reassess the clinical exam because normalization of the acute phase serum markers will not be a valid marker of disease response. When both corticosteroids and TCZ are used concomitantly, resolution of symptoms and normalization of the clinical exam suggest the prednisone dosage can be tapered and, if improvement persists, ultimately discontinued. TCZ therapy should be maintained for 1 year. Patients should be prescribed proton pump inhibitors, calcium, and vitamin D as well.

- Giant cell arteritis is the most common primary arteritis in patients older than age 50 years.
- Giant cell arteritis can cause a rapidly sequential, bilateral blindness.
- Headache is the most common initial symptom.
- Jaw claudication affects only 34%; 20% have no systemic symptoms.
- The ESR is normal in 17% of patients; CRP is a more sensitive marker.
- Treatment is warranted, even in patients likely to have some degree of intolerance to steroids, when diagnosis is nearly certain.
- Tocilizumab, an IL-6 receptor blocker, is FDA approved and has been shown to lessen total steroid dosage and duration of steroid treatment.
- Tocilizumab will produce a rapid decline in CRP and ESR, so clinical monitoring is imperative because normalization of acute phase reactants does not correlate with disease remission.

Further Reading

Dasgupta B, Borg FA, Hassan N, et al. BSR and BHPR guidelines for the management of giant cell arteritis. *Rheumatology*. 2010;49:1594–1597.

Hoffman GS. Giant cell arteritis. *Ann Intern Med*. 2016;165: ITC65–ITC79.

Hunder GG, Bloch DA, Michel BA, et al. The American College of Rheumatology 1990 criteria for the classification of giant cell arteritis. *Arthritis Rheum*. 1990;33:1122–1128.

Melson MR, Weyand CM, Newman NJ, Biousse V. The diagnosis of giant cell arteritis. *Rev Neurol Dis*. 2007;4:128–142.

Rodriguez-Valverde V, Sarabia JM, Gonzales-Gay MA, et al. Risk factors and predictive models of giant cell arteritis in polymyalgia rheumatica. *Am J Med*. 1997;102:331–336.

Smetana GW, Shmerling R. Does this patient have temporal arteritis? *JAMA*. 2002; 287(1):92–101.

Stone JH, Tuckwell K, Dimonoco S, et al. Efficacy and safety of tocilizumab in patients with giant cell arteritis: Primary and secondary outcomes from a phase 3, randomized, double-blind, placebo-controlled trial [abstract]. *Arthritis Rheumatol*. 2016;68(Suppl 10).

5 Spontaneous Cervicocerebral Artery Dissections

You are called to the emergency department to consult on a 32-year-old man who was seen the previous day complaining of 2 days of left periorbital throbbing pain, without associated nausea, vomiting, or photo- or phonophobia. He has a prior history of episodic migraine without aura but says this headache "feels different." Computed tomography (CT) of the brain obtained yesterday was normal. The patient reports he had transient relief following the "migraine cocktail" of intravenous ketorolac, diphenhydramine, and metoclopramide given yesterday but that the headache returned several hours post discharge. His exam reveals a left-sided ptosis and miosis.

What do you do now?

This patient needs to be more thoroughly evaluated. Despite the positive prior migraine history, normal imaging, and partial response to antimigraine therapies, his current headaches do not meet the criteria for migraine. Furthermore, the change in headache characteristics and the abnormal findings on his neurological examination strongly suggest a secondary headache disorder (Box 5.1). Horner syndrome can be seen in cluster headache, but this patient's symptoms are not consistent with any of the trigeminal autonomic cephalalgias.

Cervicocerebral arterial dissections (CAD) are a not uncommon but frequently underrecognized cause of severe headache associated with neurological disturbances in young patients. CAD can involve the extracranial or intracranial portions of the carotid or vertebral arteries. Dissections of the internal carotid arteries are approximately three times more common than those affecting the vertebrals. Dissections most commonly involve the extracranial portion of the artery, and the cervical segment is most often affected. Spontaneous dissections may arise from an underlying arteriopathy resulting from an unidentified connective tissue disorder. Conditions reported to be associated with these spontaneous dissections include Marfan and Behçet syndromes, Ehlers–Danlos type IV, osteogenesis imperfecta type I, fibromuscular dysplasia, autosomal dominant polycystic kidney

---

BOX 5.1 **Secondary Headache Considerations: SSNOOPPP**

Systemic symptoms: Fever, weight loss, myalgias, arthralgias, nuchal rigidity

Secondary risk factors: Cancer, HIV, immunosuppressant use

Neurologic signs/symptoms: Mental status changes, motor/sensory deficits, aphasia, reflex asymmetry, cranial nerve abnormalities (anisocoria, papilledema, Horner syndrome)

Onset: Thunderclap; during or immediately following exertion, coughing, straining, or sexual activity; following head or neck trauma

Older age: Headaches beginning or changing after age 50 years

Prior headache history: Change in pattern

Progressive worsening

Positional onset

Adapted from Dodick (2010).

---

disease, α-1 antitrypsin deficiency, and reversible cerebral vasoconstriction syndrome.

Clinically, carotid dissection may present in several ways. Headache is usually the inaugural symptom, occasionally associated with neck pain. The pain usually begins gradually but occasionally presents with a thunderclap onset. Head pain is almost always ipsilateral to the dissection but may be reported to occur as a bifrontal or global headache. Face, ear, and eye pain may accompany the headache, and approximately one-fourth of patients with spontaneous dissections report ipsilateral neck pain. The headaches are usually steady and constant; approximately 25% describe a throbbing quality. Pain severity ranges from mild discomfort to incapacitating.

In a significant minority of patients (45%), the headache of carotid dissection usually precedes the other associated symptoms. Retinal or cerebral ischemia is the most common symptom associated with carotid dissection and may present as visual obscurations and scintillations, amaurosis fugax, transient ischemic attacks, and stroke. Partial Horner syndrome is the most frequent sign of carotid dissection, occurring in as many as 58% of patients. Other associated symptoms include pulsatile tinnitus, syncope, cranial nerve palsies, and dysgeusia.

Patients with vertebral artery dissections usually present clinically with severe occipital–nuchal pain as the initial manifestation. Pain is often followed by posterior circulation symptoms such as dizziness or vertigo, dysarthria, diplopia, and ataxia. Cerebellar and lateral medullary strokes and rarely spinal cord infarctions may occur.

Although these types of dissections are classified as spontaneous to distinguish them from traumatic dissections, they often follow some "triggering" event. Spontaneous dissections have been reported to occur after vomiting, chiropractic manipulation, sporting events without associated trauma, scuba diving, sexual intercourse, vigorous coughing or sneezing, riding roller coasters or other amusement park rides, and going to the hairdresser.

Although conventional angiography has long been considered the gold standard for establishing the diagnosis of carotid dissection, noninvasive imaging techniques have become the preferred first step in diagnosis, with angiography used in younger patients when there is a high clinical suspicion for dissection not seen with noninvasive imaging procedures. Brain magnetic resonance imaging (MRI) with fat saturation and MR angiography

(MRA) and cranial CT with CT angiography (CTA) have been reported to have similar sensitivity and specificity for establishing the diagnosis. Angiographic evidence of dissection is characterized by the presence of a "string sign," a double lumen, or internal flaps. If the dissection involves the subadventitial layer of the vessel so that there is no narrowing of the lumen, angiography may miss the diagnosis, although both MRI and MRA are especially useful in diagnosing subadventitial dissections.

The pathognomonic finding of the intramural hematoma is the crescent sign, a crescentric hyperdensity surrounding a hypodense arterial lumen on T1-weighted, fat-saturated MRI (Figure 5.1), or with a suboccipital rim with an increase in vessel wall thickness but not in the lumen on CTA.

Ultrasonography [carotid duplex or transcranial Doppler (TCD)], although the least invasive imaging modality, is best used as a screening tool for dissections. Because these techniques cannot penetrate bone, they can only identify dissections more proximally, within the cervical segments of the carotid and vertebral arteries. Ultrasound findings in dissection consist of a "double lumen" sign, and TCD reveals decreased velocities in the carotid bulb and a high-resistance flow pattern in the distal arteries.

Upon establishing the diagnosis, treatment is aimed at preventing stroke. Guidelines suggest that for patients with an extracranial dissection, treatment with antiplatelet therapy should begin following diagnosis, although

(a)   (b)

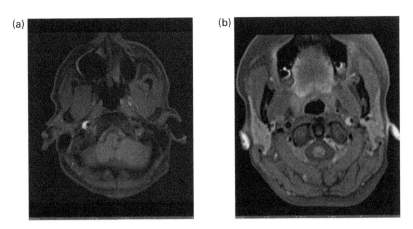

FIGURE 5.1 Crescent sign. (Courtesy of Matthew Young, DO, Department of Neuroradiology, NYU Langone Health.)

evidence for this recommendation is considered grade 2C. Noninvasive monitoring with MRA, CTA, and ultrasonography is also recommended.

Our patient had a new-onset headache with an ipsilateral partial Horner syndrome. This painful Horner strongly suggests an extracranial carotid dissection. The negative CT scan does not rule out dissection. Noninvasive imaging techniques should be used first; if negative or equivocal, the high clinical suspicion and the patient's young age mandate that conventional angiogram should be performed.

KEY POINTS TO REMEMBER

- Arterial dissections are a not uncommon but frequently underrecognized cause of headache and neurological disturbances in young patients.
- Dissections most commonly involve the extracranial portion of the artery, with the cervical segment of the carotid and the V3 segment at the C1–C2 level of the vertebral artery most often affected.
- A painful Horner syndrome should suggest the possibility of a silent carotid dissection until proven otherwise.
- Noninvasive imaging modalities (MRA/CTA) have replaced catheter angiography as preferred diagnostic tools.
- Antiplatelet therapy is recommended in cases of extracranial dissections without ischemic symptoms to prevent carotid thrombosis and embolism.

Further Reading

Dodick DW. Headache: *Pearls Semin Neurol*. 2010;30:74–81.

Liebeskind DS. Spontaneous cerebral and cervical artery dissection: Treatment and prognosis. In: Kasner SE, ed. *UpToDate*. Waltham, MA: Wolters Kluwer; 2019. https://www.uptodate.com

Schievink WI. Spontaneous dissection of the carotid and vertebral arteries. *N Engl J Med*. 2001;344:898–906.

Shakir HJ, Davies JM, Shallwani H, Siddiqui AH, Levy EI. Carotid and vertebral dissection imaging. *Curr Pain Headache Rep*. 2016;20:68–76.

Thanvi B, Munshi SK, Dawson SL, Robinson TG. Carotid and vertebral artery dissection syndromes. *Postgrad Med J*. 2005;81:383–388.

6 Chiari Malformation and Migraine

Specialties: Neurology, Radiology, and Neurosurgery

A 42-year-old woman with a long-standing history of headaches presents for evaluation. She explains that she has two headache types. The first has been present for many years, suggestive of migraine. She has never sought medical care before for these headaches because they had been relatively infrequent, occurring about once or twice a month, and until recently responded to over-the-counter products. However, during the past year, the headache severity and frequency have gradually increased, and she finds that headaches now present every waking moment. She adds that the pain is holocephalic and exacerbated by bending over to tie her shoes and Valsalva maneuvers. She has had to stop going to the gym because lifting weights and running will also worsen her baseline pain. It is for evaluation of these new daily headaches that she presents for an appointment. Although her medical and neurological examinations are normal, you order magnetic resonance imaging (MRI), which reveals a Chiari malformation type I (CMI) (Figure 6.1). At follow-up, the patient informs you that she has consulted with a neurosurgeon, who recommended surgery. The patient asks for your advice regarding the procedure.

What do you do now?

Chiari malformations are congenital deformities that are thought to arise from intrauterine underdevelopment of the posterior cranial fossa. The resultant crowding of the posterior fossa causes a downward displacement of the cerebellar tonsils through the foramen magnum and into the upper cervical spinal canal. In CMI, the tonsils extend at below the level of the foramen magnum (although a specific amount of tonsillar protrusion is not defined, at least 5 mm of descent is often cited as meeting criteria). In CMII, there is descent of the cerebellar tonsils, the cerebellar inferior vermis, and portions of the cerebellar hemispheres into the spinal canal, along with displacement of the brainstem and fourth ventricle. The most frequent form of Chiari malformation is CMII, which is associated with spina bifida and hydrocephalus. Although the exact prevalence of CMI is unknown, it is believed to be a rare disorder, affecting less than 1% of the population, with a slight female predominance.

Many patients with CMI are asymptomatic, where the deformity is an incidental finding and requires no further specific treatment. When symptomatic, clinical features usually present after age 30 years. Headache is the most common symptom of CMI, although other symptoms include dizziness, diplopia, dysphagia, nausea, weakness, and ataxia. Pain localization is often occipital–nuchal but may be generalized. Approximately 30% of patients with CMI report headaches that are precipitated by Valsalva maneuvers such as sneezing, laughing, straining, lifting, or bending over,

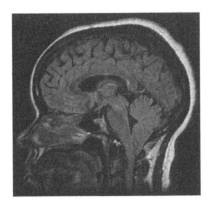

FIGURE 6.1   Chiari malformation. (Courtesy of Gordon Heller, MD, Department of Neuro-Radiology, Roosevelt Hospital Center, New York, NY.)

and approximately 20% of CMI patients experience cough headache (see Chapter 11). These cough-induced headaches are characterized by sudden-onset, short-lasting (seconds to minutes), sharp or stabbing pains of moderate to severe intensity, without associated features. Consequently, when a patient presents with a new headache meeting criteria for cough headache, an MRI brain should be done to evaluate the posterior fossa. Also, CMI can be associated with headaches that last up to several days and rarely may cause a continuous headache of fluctuating intensity.

It has been postulated that the Valsalva and cough headaches associated with CMI may be the result of transient pressure dissociation between the intracranial and intraspinal compartments that causes the cerebellar tonsils to further extend through the foramen magnum, producing pain via traction and pressure on pain-sensitive structures. The pathophysiological correlates of the other headache subtypes are not known. Some investigators believe that the occipitonuchal headaches are also the result of tonsillar descent (see Pasqual et al., 1992), but others have found no relationship between the descent of the tonsils and the presence or absence of headache (see Stovner, 1993).

Our patient is suffering from migraine headaches. She reports no history of occipitonuchal, Valsalva, or cough headaches. The headache of CMI is by definition a secondary headache, and it is not causally linked to migraine or other primary headaches. In the various reviews of headache and CMI, the prevalence of migraine and tension-type headaches was similar to that of the general population. Because many CMI patients are asymptomatic, they are identified only when they have a neuroimaging procedure done for another reason. Because migraine is so common, the co-occurrence of the two disorders will occur by chance in many people, as it has in our patient. In these asymptomatic patients, there is no indication for a suboccipital craniotomy. Even when patients have headache symptoms consistent with CMI, the indication for suboccipital craniotomy is not clear, and further workup to confirm obstruction of cerebrospinal fluid (CSF) flow must be done before proceeding. The clinical features of a headache secondary to CMI can sometimes overlap with migraine, which can also make it difficult to sort out. Spontaneous intracranial hypotension can often present with cerebellar tonsil descent resembling CMI, and for that reason MRI brain should be done with and without contrast. If surgery is undertaken, among other things, complications of surgery include recurrent infection and the formation of fluid accumulations and cysts, as well as the potential for no headache improvement in cases in which individuals may have coexistent migraine that is not being addressed. Attempting treatment with medications that can lower CSF pressure and help migraine, such as acetazolamide, topiramate, or even indomethacin, is a reasonable first step in cases in which the diagnosis remains unclear.

KEY POINTS TO REMEMBER

- Headaches with CMI are the most common symptom.
- Headaches with CMI are usually occipitonuchal.
- Headaches with CMI worsen with Valsalva maneuvers, especially coughing.
- Headaches with CMI result from transient pressure dissociation between the intracranial and intraspinal compartments, causing increased tonsillar descent through the foramen magnum.
- Headaches with CMI may co-occur in patients with migraine or tension-type headache but are not causal of these primary headaches.

Further Reading

Langridge B, Phillips E, Choi D. Chiari malformation type 1: A systematic review of natural history and conservative management. *World Neurosurg.* 2017;104:213–219.

Meadows J, Kraut M, Guarnieri M, et al. Asymptomatic Chiari type I malformations identified on magnetic resonance imaging. *J Neurosurg.* 2000;92:920–926.

Pasqual J, Oterino A, Berciano J. Headache in type I Chiari malformation. *Neurology.* 1992;42:1519–1521.

Riveira C, Pasqual J. Is Chiari type I malformation a reason for chronic daily headache? *Curr Pain Headache Rep.* 2007;11:53–55.

Stovner LJ. Headache associated with the Chiari type I malformation. *Headache.* 1993;33:175–181.

7 New Daily Persistent Headache

A 31-year-old man is referred by his primary care physician and a local pain clinic due to persistent headaches. He is vague as to the nature of the pain and states that the location is "basically all over" and is rated as moderate in intensity. He is clear about the onset of pain, however: It began on a specific date last winter, during which he thinks he had an upper respiratory virus. He states that the upper respiratory symptoms of cough and nasal congestion dissipated after 5 days; however, the headache has been persistent and constant. At times, he does become slightly sensitive to bright lights and prefers being in a dark quiet room. He can also have associated mild nausea. He cannot identify any triggers or exacerbating factors and emphasizes that he "just wants to have a pain-free day." He denies a significant history of headache. He has remained intractable to many preventive and acute medications. His mood has been suffering as well, and he just started working with a therapist for depression. Medical history and examination are unremarkable.

What do you do now?

New daily persistent headache (NDPH) is a rare primary headache disorder characterized by persistent headache with a particular profile because it starts one day with a clearly remembered onset and continues in a daily pattern. NDPH predominantly affects individuals without a history of prior headache. However, patients with prior episodic headache are not excluded from NDPH diagnosis if NDPH is different from the previous headache and they do not endorse an increasing headache frequency prior to onset or associated with medication overuse. It is very often disabling and may significantly affect the individual's quality of life and can lead to psychiatric conditions. Often, patients can recall a viral-type illness just preceding the onset of the headaches, but this is not universal. The patient described seems to fit the category well, including NDPH's notorious resistance to treatment.

The most important first step in cases such as this is to exclude secondary causes, particularly treatable ones, such as neoplastic disease, cerebral vasculitis, cerebral venous thrombosis, chronic sinusitis (particularly sphenoid sinusitis, which may have a paucity of "sinus" symptoms), idiopathic intracranial hypertension (pseudotumor cerebri, which of course may present without the usual papilledema), low cerebrospinal fluid (CSF) pressure headache syndrome, and cervical arterial or spinal disease. Treatable systemic illness, such as endocrinological disease, chronic infections, or collagen vascular disease, can also lead to daily headache. Less treatable mimics of NDPH include post-traumatic headache and post meningitis headache (Box 7.1).

Diagnostic investigation in this patient should therefore probably include magnetic resonance imaging of the brain before and after gadolinium;

BOX 7.1 **ICHD-3 Diagnostic Criteria for New Daily Persistent Headache**

A. Persistent headache fulfilling criteria B and C
B. Distinct and clearly remembered onset, with pain becoming continuous and unremitting within 24 hours
C. Present for >3 months
D. Not better accounted for by another ICHD-3 diagnosis

ICHD-3, *International Classification of Headache Disorders*, third edition.

lumbar puncture with measurement of opening pressure and CSF analysis for infectious or inflammatory causes; and systemic screening for infectious and inflammatory disease, including erythrocyte sedimentation rate, Lyme titer, lupus testing, VDRL, complete blood count, and serum chemistry screening. Thyroid screening, as well as screening for diabetes, is sensible if there are suggestive features. (This patient was tachycardic—perhaps related to a hyperthyroid state.)

Regarding the etiology of NDPH, this is entirely unclear. The fact that many cases can be traced to a viral illness suggests that an infectious process may have altered head nociceptive physiology in some way (similar to a suggested etiology for the fibromyalgia syndrome). A significant fraction of patients with NDPH have Epstein–Barr viral antibodies, denoting previous infection. But a previous or preceding viral infection might simply be coincidental. Rozen and Swiden (2007) found that CSF tumor necrosis factor-α (TNF-α) levels were increased in all of a group of NDPH patients, suggestive of central nervous system inflammation. (Interestingly, TNF-α levels were also increased in their control group consisting of chronic migraine and post-traumatic headache patients). It has also been postulated that cervical spine joint hypermobility may be a predisposing factor for the development of NDPH as well. Or could NDPH simply represent a subtype of chronic migraine or chronic tension-type headache with more abrupt onset than usual? It is hoped that these issues will be sorted out as reliable biochemical, imaging, and other markers for the primary headaches emerge.

Treatment of NDPH is generally never fully effective (another good reason to search for a treatable cause). In clinical practice, most headache specialists treat NDPH based on the prominent headache phenotype, whether migrainous or tension-type. Virtually all prophylactic agents have been tried, with varying results, including tricyclic antidepressants, selective serotonin reuptake inhibitors, beta-blockers, calcium channel blockers, antiepileptic drugs (particularly gabapentin, topiramate, and valproate), antispasmodics, and muscle relaxants. Intravenous dihydroergotamine has been proposed as a several-day course to interrupt the cycle of daily headaches and has been successful in some cases. This could be of use in the patient here, along with the institution of a novel prophylactic agent, perhaps in the anticonvulsant category. Botulinum toxin has been tried anecdotally in a number of cases of NDPH, with mixed results. Calcitonin gene-related peptide monoclonal antibodies could certainly be tried as well, although currently there are no data to support what impact they may have.

Medication overuse is frequently a problem, for obvious reasons, and must be dealt with in order to have a chance at successful outcome. With patients such as the one summarized here, it is important to stress the importance of nonpharmacological pain-reducing techniques such as relaxation training and lifestyle adjustment (sleep regulation, regular exercise, etc.) and to remain optimistic about continuing the search for the best prophylactic program, which may include polypharmacy. Counseling can be important when patients become demoralized. Procedures such as occipital nerve blocks and/or neuromodulation may have promise but remain unproven. Some cases do remit on their own.

KEY POINTS TO REMEMBER

- New daily persistent headache can have either chronic migraine or chronic tension-type headache features. Only a sudden onset and persistence are required for the diagnosis of NDPH.
- A number of occult mimics must be ruled out in these cases despite the benign appearance of most patients.
- There may be two clinical subtypes: a self-limited form and a refractory persistent form.
- Treatment is unsatisfactory in most patients, although some degree of pain reduction is almost always achievable.

Further Reading

Rozen T. New daily persistent headache: An update. *Curr Pain Headache Rep.* 2014;18:431.

Rozen T, Swiden SZ. Elevation of CSF tumor necrosis factor levels in new daily persistent headache and treatment refractory chronic migraine. *Headache.* 2007;47:1050–1055.

Spears RC. Efficacy of botulinum toxin type A in new daily persistent headache. *J Headache Pain.* 2008;9(6):405–406.

Yamani N, Olesen J. New daily persistent headache: A systematic review on an enigmatic disorder. *J Headache Pain.* 2019;20:80.

8   Spontaneous Intracranial Hypotension

A 50-year-old woman presents with a 3-week headache that began without a known precipitating event. The headache began soon after awakening one morning and has persisted until now. This headache is global and throbbing, of moderate severity, and associated with neck pain and stiffness. The headache is strictly positional in that it worsens with standing and resolves when she lays down. Her exam is entirely normal, and there is no evidence of orthostatic blood pressure or pulse changes. A lumbar puncture, done in the lateral decubitus position, reveals an opening pressure of 170 mm H_2O (normal: 100–180 mm H_2O). Contrast-enhanced magnetic resonance imaging (MRI) of the brain is normal.

What do you do now?

This patient describes a new-onset headache that is notable for its orthostatic features. Causes of orthostatic headaches include postdural puncture headaches (see Chapter 23), postural orthostatic tachycardia syndrome, cervicogenic headache (see Chapter 13), diabetes insipidus, and new daily persistent headache (see Chapter 7). Postural headaches may also occur with migraine and may result from posterior decompression surgery used in the treatment of Chiari malformations (see Chapter 6). This disorder should be included in the differential diagnosis of any patient who complains of new onset of daily persistent headaches, as well as patients with refractory daily headache, especially if there is a positional element.

Spontaneous intracranial hypotension (SIH) is a well-recognized syndrome that is characterized by orthostatic headaches in association with a variety of other symptoms. SIH, by definition, begins without an identifiable precipitant. The syndrome is caused by an occult leakage of cerebrospinal fluid (CSF) through weakness of the dura from nerve root sleeves, dural rents caused by herniated discs or osteophytic microspurs, or by CSF-venous fistulas. These entities produce a decrease in CSF volume but not necessarily a decrease in CSF pressure.

The exact incidence of SIH is not known; it may be underrecognized by many clinicians, especially when the patient presents with long-standing symptoms. Often, the diagnosis is made accidentally when a patient with daily headaches is found to have features of SIH on the MRI. In the majority of cases, the cause of SIH is unclear, but possible precipitants include a history of trivial trauma and weakness of the dural sac. The traumatic event is typically minor and includes coughing, straining, sexual activity, lifting, bending, minor falls, sports injuries, and gardening. The dural sac weakness may be the result of connective tissue disorders (Marfan and Ehlers–Danlos syndromes) or meningeal diverticula; in fact, 16–38% of patients with SIH are noted to have connective tissue disorders.

The characteristic clinical feature of SIH is headache. The typical headache is positional in that the pain worsens with sitting or standing and lessens with recumbency. The longer the patient remains upright, the longer it takes for the headache to dissipate when lying down. The headaches are usually throbbing, bilateral, and worsened by Valsalva maneuvers. Although this orthostatic headache is classic for this syndrome, other non-orthostatic presentations are possible. Also, a previously orthostatic headache may become chronic and unremitting over time, losing the positionality. The headaches may be associated with neck stiffness, tinnitus, hypacusia, photophobia, intrascapular pain, nausea, vomiting, blurred vision, and diplopia (secondary to cranial nerve palsies).

Leaks of CSF in SIH are usually found in the thoracic spine but at times are seen at the cervical or lumbar levels. These leaks frequently occur along the dural root sleeves, and meningeal diverticula are often located in the thoracic and upper lumbar spine. The leakage of CSF results in a decrease in the total CSF volume, which causes sinking of the brain in the skull. This "brain sag" induces traction on the pain-sensitive suspending and anchoring structures of the brain and is responsible for the headache and associated signs and symptoms of this disorder. The positional component of the headache is the result of the increase in the downward displacement of the brain and the increase in traction upon the pain-sensitive structures that occurs in a gravity-dependent manner when the patient assumes an upright position. Traction upon cranial nerves III–VIII and the brainstem results in nerve palsies and mental status changes, whereas the changes in pressure that are transmitted into the perilymphatic fluid produce the tinnitus, hypacusia, and vestibular complaints.

The diagnosis of SIH may be established in several ways, but unfortunately there is not a single modality that consistently reveals the answer. Patients may require several tests to establish the diagnosis. In some, no identifiable abnormality is uncovered. Brain MRI with and without gadolinium should be the initial test in the workup of SIH. Noncontrast MRI may demonstrate brain sag, descent of the cerebellar tonsils (pseudo-Chiari I), a decrease in the prepontine or perichiasmatic cisterns, flattening of the optic chiasm, posterior fossa crowding, a decrease in the size of the ventricles, subdural collections, and enlargement of the venous sinuses. Contrast-enhanced MRI typically shows diffuse pachymeningeal, but not leptomeningeal, enhancement. Pachymeningeal enhancement is not always present and may disappear over time; therefore, it is not required for the diagnosis. In fact, a negative brain MRI does not rule out SIH. In a study of patients with documented SIH, dural enhancement was seen in 83%, brain sag in 61%, and venous distension in 75% (Kranz et al. 2017).

Computed tomographic myelography and heavily T2-weighted MRI of the spine are both potentially useful imaging tools to identify the cause of the leak. MRI is often used first because it is a less invasive procedure; however, CT myelography is better at visualizing slow-flow leaks, evaluating calcified disk herniations, and identifying CSF-venous fistulas (Krantz et al. 2017). Spine MRI may demonstrate extra-arachnoid fluid collections, meningeal diverticula, pachymeningeal enhancement (usually cervical), and engorgement of the spinal epidural venous plexus. CT myelography can also demonstrate the site of the CSF leak as evidenced by extradural contrast extravasation, meningeal diverticula, or extra-arachnoid collections of CSF.

When SIH is the result of a rapid-flow leak, identification of the site of the leak may be ascertained by dynamic CT myelography or digital subtraction myelography. Dynamic CT myelography is performed by imaging the spine with high-speed CT following intrathecal contrast administration, but without the myelography.

According to the *International Classification of Headache Disorders*, third edition, criteria, the opening pressure in patients with SIH is usually very low (≤ 60 mm H_2O), yet recent evidence suggests this is not always the case. Normal pressures are seen in approximately 40% of patients with SIH, and high opening pressures (>200 mm H_2O) have been reported in patients with active leaks. The CSF is usually normal but may show elevated protein, white blood cell, or red blood cell counts. In general, lumbar puncture is not performed early in the workup of SIH because it may worsen the clinical picture and because removing fluid may cause pachymeningeal enhancement on MRI.

Treatment of SIH includes conservative measures such as bed rest and hydration and caffeine administration (by mouth or intravenously). Epidural blood patching, in which the patient is injected with 10–20 cc of autologous blood in the lumbar epidural region, may provide relief. Some patients require repeated blood patches for relief. Success rates for the first patch range from 36% to 90%, and the efficacy of each subsequent patch is approximately 30%. Approximately half of the patients who do not respond to the first or second patch will respond to additional patches. Success rates are enhanced if the patches are targeted to the site of leakage that was demonstrated on cisternography or myelography. If repeated blood patches are unsuccessful and the site of the leak is known, percutaneous placement of 4–20 mL of fibrin sealant injected via a transforaminal approach may offer relief. For refractory cases, surgical exploration and repair is necessary.

Our patient has clinical features of SIH, although her brain MRI and CSF pressure are normal. This does not eliminate SIH as a possibility, however, and further imaging of her spine is warranted to identify the site of the potential leak. If a leak site is identified, then targeted blood patching should be tried, followed by percutaneous fibrin injections if multiple patches are unsuccessful. If these measures fail, then surgical exploration and repair should be attempted.

If no leak is found on spinal imaging, the clinician should, before discounting SIH as the diagnosis, consider the possibility of a CSF fistula as the cause. These fistulas, usually located along thoracic nerve roots, consist of a direct, aberrant connection between the spinal subarachnoid space and a draining paraspinal vein. This anomaly causes low CSF volume by allowing the CSF to drain directly into the venous circulation. Like our patient, patients with CSF-venous fistulas report positional headaches and may have normal opening pressures and normal brain and spine imaging. Special imaging techniques such as digital subtraction myelography may identify these fistulas.

KEY POINTS TO REMEMBER

- Spontaneous intracranial hypotension results from an occult leak of CSF usually without precipitant through weakness of the dura from nerve root sleeves, dural rents caused by herniated discs or osteophytic microspurs, or by CSF-venous fistulas.
- Spontaneous intracranial hypotension may be preceded by trivial trauma.
- Some patients have a connective tissue disorder.
- Opening pressure may be below 60 mm H_2O in the sitting position, but 40% of patients have normal opening pressure.
- Contrast-enhanced MRI may demonstrate enhancement of the pachymeninges but not the leptomeninges.
- Blood patching success rates are 30–90% for the first patch but 30% for each subsequent patch, so subsequent trials should be attempted if the first fails.
- CSF-venous fistulas should be considered in cases of SIH when spinal imaging does not find a source of the leak.

Further Reading

Ferrante E, Trimboli M, Rubino F. Spontaneous intracranial hypotension: Review and expert opinion. *Acta Neurol Belg.* 2020;120:9–18.

Kranz PG, Gray L, Amrhein TJ. Spontaneous intracranial hypotension: 10 myths and misperceptions. *Headache.* 2018;58:948–959.

Kranz PG, Gray L, Malinzak MD, Amrhein TJ. Spontaneous intracranial hypotension: Pathogenesis, diagnosis and treatment. *Neuroimag Clin North Am.* 2019;29:581–594.

Kranz PG, Malinzak MD, Amrhein TJ, Gray L. Update on the diagnosis and treatment of spontaneous intracranial hypotension. *Curr Pain Headache Rep.* 2017;21:37.

Schievink WI, Moser FG, Maya MM, Prasad RS. Digital subtraction myelography for the identification of spontaneous spinal CSF-venous fistulas. *J Neurosurg Spine.* 2016;24:960–964.

9 Migraine with Persistent Aura

Specialties: Neurology, Ophthalmology, and Emergency Medicine

A 65-year-old woman with a history of migraine with visual aura since her twenties reports that 7 days ago, she developed her typical headache that was preceded by scintillating scotoma in her left visual field. Prior to this episode, she had not had any episodes of visual aura in more than a decade, although she experiences migraine attacks approximately once per month. That aura, like all of her previous, occurred spontaneously, lasted 30 minutes, and was followed by a right-sided, throbbing headache. The migraine headache pain resolved within 1 hour of treatment with rizatriptan; however, the aura recurred soon after and has been fluctuating in size but never completely disappearing. The headache has not recurred, and she has not had any other neurological symptoms. She has no other medical problems and is on no other medication. Computed tomography of the head is normal. An ophthalmological evaluation was normal, as was an electroencephalography. The patient is quite disabled by the visual phenomena and has been afraid to drive her car for the past week. She is very worried that she has had a stroke.

What do you do now?

Approximately 20% of individuals with migraine experience an aura with their attacks. Auras are characterized by transient episodes of fully reversible focal neurological disturbances that may precede or accompany the headache onset. Occasionally, auras may occur without headache. In general, auras develop gradually over 5–20 minutes and resolve within 1 hour or less. The migraine aura may manifest as a visual, sensory, or language disturbance and may be simple or complex (Box 9.1). The *International Classification of Headache Disorders*, third edition (ICHD-3), classification of migraine with aura (Box 9.2) provides specific details to make the diagnosis. When motor weakness occurs as part of an aura, the diagnosis of familial or sporadic hemiplegic migraine should be considered.

BOX 9.1 **Migraine Auras**

Visual
Photopsias
Phosphenes
Scotomata
Geometric shapes
Fortification spectra
Micro-/macropsia
Mosaic vision
Metamorphopsia
Sensory
Paresthesias
Cheiro-oral numbness
Olfactory/gustatory/auditory hallucinations
Speech
Dysphasic
Dysarthric
Aphasic

BRAINSTEM

Dyarthria
Vertigo
Tinnitus
Hyperacusis
Diplopia
Ataxia not attributable to a sensory deficit

Most auras are of a visual nature and may present as photopsias or *phosphenes* (unformed flashes of lights), geometric forms, shimmering waves, or scotoma (positive or negative). Visual auras are usually bilateral and slowly move across the visual field. The classic visual aura, the fortification spectrum, is characterized by a zigzag or herringbone pattern at the point of visual fixation. Over time, this shape enlarges to encroach upon the visual hemifield, assuming a jagged, convex shape. The borders of the spectrum typically are shimmering, composed of flashing lights, jagged lines, or geometric patterns that surround a blind spot (*scotoma*) that may occupy the center of the design. *Metamorphopsia* is an abnormality in visual perception in which the shapes or borders of objects become distorted or disjointed. Patients who have metamorphoptic auras often report that objects appear smaller (*micropsia*) or larger (*macropsia*) than they really are. These patients may note that objects appear to be farther away (*telopsia*). Other common auras include sensory disturbances (paresthesias and numbness). The typical sensory aura, cheiro-oral numbness, is characterized by paresthesias that begin in the hand, slowly march upward to involve the forearm, and then produce numbness of the ipsilateral face, lip, and chin. Language disturbances usually manifest as dysphasic speech; true aphasia is very rare.

Rarely, the migraine aura may persist for extended periods of time. The ICHD-3 designates two subclasses of prolonged aura. When one or more aura symptoms continue for more than 1 hour and there is evidence of an ischemic lesion in the appropriate site on neuroimaging, the diagnosis of migrainous infarction is used. If the aura symptoms persist for more than 1 week without radiographic evidence of a stroke, then the diagnosis is persistent aura without infarction. Patients suffering from very prolonged auras, in which aura symptoms recur repeatedly on a daily basis or persist unabated for months or years, have been described and are often referred to as being in "migraine aura status."

Obviously, any patient who suffers from a prolonged neurological deficit requires a complete workup, including neuroimaging, to rule out cerebrovascular disease. Other disorders that may mimic prolonged auras include occipital lobe epilepsy; vertebrobasilar transient ischemic attacks; posterior leukoencephalopathy; carotid or vertebral artery dissection (see Chapter 5); retinal detachment; hematological diseases (polycythemia vera); hyperhomocysteinemia; mitochondrial encephalopathy, lactic acidosis, and stroke-like episodes MELAS syndrome; and cerebral autosomal dominant arteriopathy with subcortical infarcts and leukoencephalopathy (CADASIL).

Our patient has had a continuous visual aura for the past week. Although her neurological examination is normal, we must order magnetic resonance imaging (MRI) of the brain, to rule out secondary mimics such as infarction or posterior leukoencephalopathy, and blood work, to screen for blood

---

BOX 9.3 **Treatment of Prolonged Auras**

OLDER THERAPIES

Inhalation of 10% CO_2 and 90% O_2
Inhalation of amyl nitrate
Inhalation of isoproterenol
Sublingual nifedipine 10 mg

NEWER THERAPIES (BASED ON CORTICAL SPREADING DEPRESSION MODEL)

intravenous furosemide 20 mg
Oral acetazolamide 500–750 mg daily
Intranasal ketamine 25 mg
Intravenous prochlorperazine 10 mg q 8 hours with magnesium sulfate 1 g q 12 hours
Single-pulse transcranial magnetic stimulation, 4 pulses twice daily and as needed, up to 17 pulses per day

Source: Rozen (2003).

---

dyscrasias, increased homocysteine levels, and autoimmune disorders. A transcranial Doppler can also be helpful looking for evidence of a shunt. Because her visual disturbances are apparently in both eyes, dissection is unlikely. A normal MRI would essentially rule out CADASIL. This patient seems to meet the criteria for persistent aura without infarction.

There is no standard treatment protocol for patients suffering from prolonged auras (Box 9.3). Older therapies reported to demonstrate success in individual patients include inhalation therapy with 10% carbon dioxide and 90% oxygen, amyl nitrate or isoproterenol, and sublingual nifedipine. These treatments were based on the theory that migrainous auras were the result of prolonged vasoconstriction. Aura is now believed to be the result of cortical spreading depression, and treatments aimed at interfering with this mechanism include intravenous furosemide, magnesium sulfate and prochlorperazine, and intranasal ketamine. Oral divalproex, acetazolamide, verapamil, flunarizine, lamotrigine, gabapentin, and memantine have also been reported to be beneficial. Some patients find single-pulse transcranial magnetic stimulation to be helpful. Because aura is considered a stroke risk factor, managing aura, as well as other vascular risk factors, is important.

- Migraine aura occurs in approximately 20% of individuals with migraine and is usually a visual, sensory, or language disturbance.
- Motor auras are not typical of migraine.
- Migraine aura develops over 5–20 minutes and resolves within 1 hour or less.
- Rarely, auras persist for extended periods of time; these are divided as follows:

  Migrainous infarction: When one or more aura symptoms continue for more than 1 hour and there is evidence of an ischemic lesion in the appropriate site on neuroimaging.

  Persistent aura without infarction: Aura symptoms persisting for more than 1 week without radiographic evidence of a stroke.

Further Reading

Agostini E, Aliprandi A. Complications of migraine with aura. *Neurol Sci.* 2006;27:S91–S95.

Evans RW, Burch RC, Frishberg BM, et al. Neuroimaging for migraine: The American Headache Society systematic review and evidence-based guideline. *Headache.* 2020;60(2):318–336.

Rozen TD. Aborting a prolonged migrainous aura with intravenous prochlorperazine and magnesium sulfate. *Headache.* 2003;43:901–903.

Schankin CJ, Viana M, Goadsby PJ. Persistent and repetitive visual disturbances in migraine: A review. *Headache.* 2017; 57:1–16.

Tietjen GE, Maly EF. Migraine and ischemic stroke in women: A narrative review. *Headache.* 2020;60(5):843–863.

van Dongen RM, Haan J. Symptoms related to the visual system in migraine. *F1000Res.* 2019 (July 30);8:F1000 Faculty Rev-1219. doi:10.12688/f1000research.18768.1

10 Vestibular Migraine

A 32-year-old woman describes recurring bouts of severe disabling vertigo. Episodes can be as brief as 5 minutes and as long as 4 or 5 hours. During spells, she is often nauseated, although rarely vomits, and tends to be sensitive to light and sound, seeking a quiet dark place and keeping her head very still. She has had bitemporal headaches with a few of these spells, but this is unusual. There are no other symptoms such as visual changes, weakness, paresthesias, or abnormal movements. She does find it impossible to concentrate during spells of vertigo. Meclizine has not helped acutely. An otolaryngologist has done "vestibular testing," which is normal and led to the diagnosis of "migraine." Audiometry was normal as well. Magnetic resonance imaging (MRI) of the head and electroencephalogram (EEG) are likewise normal. The one thing that has helped is high-dose lorazepam. Neurological examination is normal, except for a mildly positive Hallpike maneuver—she is very uncomfortable with extreme head turning to either side.

What do you do now?

Vertigo and migraine have a number of associations. Vertigo is a relatively common, although generally mild, aura symptom in patients with migraine with aura. A childhood syndrome believed to be closely related to migraine, benign paroxysmal vertigo of childhood, occurs in the absence of headache, although a family history of migraine is common, and these children are very likely to develop migraine. (This syndrome is characterized by recurrent brief bouts of vertigo and nausea, with intervening asymptomatic periods.) Many patients with migraine suffer from motion sickness, including the visually induced variety (e.g., watching widescreen movies). Finally, migraine with brainstem aura (MWBSA) is commonly accompanied by vertigo. MWBSA has strict criteria, however (Box 10.1), including the presence of at least two of the following aura symptoms: dysarthria, vertigo, tinnitus, reduced hearing (hypacusia), diplopia, bilateral visual field manifestations, ataxia, decreased consciousness, and bilateral limb/trunk sensation changes, each lasting only 30 minutes at most.

Recurrent vertigo without headache as a migraine subtype in adults is more controversial, but it has long been discussed in the literature. There are no known biological or clinical markers, but proposed definitions of such "vestibular migraine" (VM) generally include (1) recurrent bouts of vertigo lasting minutes to hours, (2) a current or past diagnosis of migraine, and (3) some co-occurrences of both. The current International Headache Society and Bárány Society criteria are even more strict (Box 10.2), requiring headache or clear migraine accompaniments in more than 50% of the bouts of vertigo.

How might migraine produce vertigo? This is not known, but a number of intriguing explanations have been proposed, including (1) cortical spreading depression in the region of the lateral temporal lobe (known to be a site where other pathological processes can produce vertigo), (2) migraine-induced reduction of regional blood flow involving the circulation of the inner ear, and (3) release of vasoactive peptides by trigeminal nerve endings in the vicinity of the inner ear resulting in changes in vestibular neural activity.

In evaluating patients with possible vestibular migraine, the first step is deciding if the symptoms do indeed represent true vertigo rather than lightheadedness, ataxia, or panic. This is generally not too challenging if the differences are explained to patients. Illnesses that may present with

---

BOX 10.1 **Diagnostic Criteria for Migraine with Brainstem Aura (Previously Termed Basilar-Type Migraine)**

A. Migraine with reversible neurological accompaniments with at least three of the following six characteristics:
  1. At least one aura symptom spreads gradually over approximately 5 minutes.
  2. Two or more aura symptoms occur in succession.
  3. Each individual aura symptom lasts 5–60 minutes.
  4. At least one aura symptom is unilateral.
  5. At least one aura symptom is positive.
  6. The aura is accompanied, or followed within 60 minutes, by headache.

B. Aura includes both of the following:
  1. At least two of the following fully reversible brainstem symptoms:
    a. Dysarthria
    b. Vertigo
    c. Tinnitus
    d. Hypacusis
    e. Diplopia
    f. Ataxia not attributable to sensory deficit
    g. Decreased level of consciousness
  2. No motor or retinal symptoms

Adapted from the *International Classification of Headache Disorders*, third edition.

---

episodic vertigo that can mimic migrainous vertigo include Meniere disease (MD), persistent postural–perceptual dizziness (PPPD), benign paroxysmal positional vertigo (BPPV), migraine with brainstem aura (as mentioned previously), otologic conditions such as perilymphatic fistula and semicircular canal dehiscence, demyelinating disease (with plaque(s) in the region of vestibular nuclei), transient ischemic attacks, and acoustic nerve region tumors (e.g., Schwannoma, meningioma, and epidermoid) (Table 10.1). Meniere disease eventually involves some degree of hearing loss (most commonly in the low-frequency ranges). Hearing loss is also common with acoustic nerve masses, which is much less likely in migraine. PPPD manifests with essentially constant disequilibrium rather than true vertigo, with normal neurological and otological examinations and testing. It carries the stigma of a "functional" syndrome, but although the pathophysiology is unknown, it is likely due to dysfunction in postural control

BOX 10.2   **Diagnostic Criteria for Vestibular Migraine**

A. At least five episodes fulfilling criteria C and D
B. A current or past history of migraine without aura or migraine with aura
C. Vestibular symptoms of moderate or severe intensity, lasting between 5 minutes and 72 hours
D. At least half of episodes are associated with at least one of the following three migrainous features:
  1. Headache with at least two of the following four characteristics:
    a. Unilateral location
    b. Pulsating quality
    c. Moderate or severe intensity
    d. Aggravation by routine physical activity
  2. Photophobia and phonophobia
  3. Visual aura
E. Not better accounted for by another ICHD diagnosis or by another vestibular disorder

ICHD, *International Classification of Headache Disorders.*
Adapted from ICHD-3.

mechanisms, poor cortical integration of positional input, or a combination of these. Perilymph fistula, an abnormal communication between inner and middle ear compartments, leads to fluctuating perilymph pressure and resulting effects on semicircular canals leading to tinnitus, hearing loss, and vertigo (with possible nausea). This can be due to an antecedent pressure trauma such as repeated violent coughing or sneezing, scuba diving, or lifting. Superior semicircular canal (SSC) dehiscence results from an anatomical deficiency in the roof of the SSC and leads to pressure change–induced vertigo. It is generally diagnosed on computed tomography and with electrophysiological vestibular testing. BPPV is thought to be caused by abnormal formation or location of calcium carbonate crystals (otoconia) within the semicircular canals that interfere with normal endolymph flow. In BPPV, with head position change (e.g., during Hallpike maneuver), vertigo flares, and it tends to resolve with restriction of movement. Acute labyrinthitis, or vestibular neuronitis, usually occurs as a single episode and is longer lasting than VM. Of interest is that position change may certainly trigger migraine-related vertigo, so that is not a particularly helpful clue. For unknown reasons, migraine is much more common in both MD and

TABLE 10.1 Differential Diagnosis of Recurrent Vertigo and Diagnostic Clues

Condition	Clues to Diagnosis
Migraine with brainstem aura	Migraine headaches with aura symptoms suggestive of subcortical/brainstem origin
Benign paroxysmal positional vertigo	Strictly brought on by head position change
Vestibular neuronitis/labyrinthitis	Single episode, hours to days
Meniere disease	Bouts of severe vertigo and nausea with hearing loss and/or tinnitus
Post-traumatic vertigo	History of trauma, symptoms similar to BPV
Phobic/psychogenic vertigo	Situational, history of anxiety, no nystagmus
Perilymphatic fistula	History of antecedent barotrauma, forceful nose blowing, sneeze, etc.; hearing loss
Labyrinthine or brainstem ischemia	Other signs of neurological dysfunction
Meningitis—carcinomatous, tuberculous, fungal	Other cranial nerve dysfunction, meningismus
Brainstem or cerebellopontine tumor	Hearing loss, signs of brainstem dysfunction
Complex partial seizures	History of epilepsy, abnormal EEG
Multiple sclerosis—brainstem plaque	Other neurological signs and symptoms
Medication effect—aspirin, phenytoin, aminoglycosides, cisplatin	Correlates with medication changes; constant
Vestibular migraine	History of migraine, aura, or other migraine symptoms; accompanied by headache
Persistent postural–perceptual dizziness	Constant disequilibrium rather than true vertigo, with normal neurological and otological exams

BPV, benign positional vertigo; EEG, electroencephalogram.

BPPV, so there may be causal links between these conditions or shared pathophysiological underpinnings. Finally, it is important to remember that because migraine is so common, the coincidence of migraine and vestibular disease is certainly possible without causation in either direction.

This patient may have migrainous vertigo. Although headache is not common for this patient, it does occur during some bouts of vertigo. There are no additional neurological symptoms to suggest MWBSA. There are no accompanying neurological deficits, which speaks against a destructive intracranial lesion, and this patient's evaluation has already included negative MRI, audiometry, and EEG.

Treatment of VM, when successful, can be very gratifying. Elimination of triggers (sleep deprivation, ingested substances, etc.) is very important and may serve as the key therapeutic approach. Acute attacks may respond to meclizine or dimenhydramine (Dramamine®), but as with the patient described here, these are usually not sufficient. Promethazine and metaclopramide are better in general, but frequent use can lead to unwanted side effects. Triptans have been useful for many patients when taken soon after the vertigo begins, which stands to reason, although there is no evidence to support their use. For prophylaxis, beta-blockers, calcium channel blockers, tricyclic antidepressants, clonazepam, topiramate, and lamotrigine have been successful in selected cases. In our center, we have found nortriptyline 25–50 mg qhs, topiramate 50–200 mg daily in two divided doses, and a combination of amitriptyline (5–10 mg) and chlordiazepoxide (12.5–25 mg) in the evening to be useful options. Selected patients have also responded to calcitonin gene-related peptide monoclonal antibodies.

When migraine targeted therapy fails, it is worth considering alternative explanations such as PPPD. Treatment of PPPD and Meniere disease is challenging, but vestibular rehabilitation therapy and cognitive–behavioral therapy have been very successful in selected cases. So-called "canalith repositioning" techniques that involve some form of repetitive Epley maneuvers has been shown to be helpful in BPPV but not particularly useful for vestibular migraine.

- Vestibular migraine should be considered in patients in whom other causes of recurrent vertigo have been excluded or are unlikely.
- Generally, patients with VM have a clear history of migraine and at least several occasions when migraine headache and vertigo co-occurred.
- Treatment for MV is similar to migraine headache treatment—elimination of triggers, acute treatment, and prophylactic medication.
- Persistent dizziness in the absence of headache or other migraine features is unlikely to be related to migraine and may represent vestibular pathology or PPPD.

Further Reading

Eggers, SDZ. Migraine-related vertigo: Diagnosis and treatment. *Curr Pain Headache Rep.* 2007;11:217–226.

Headache Classification Committee of the International Headache Society. The *International Classification of Headache Disorders*, 3rd edition. *Cephalalgia.* 2018;38:1–211.

Huang TC, Wang SJ, Kheradmand A. Vestibular migraine: An update on current understanding and future directions. *Cephalalgia.* 2020;40:107–121.

Staab JP, Eckhardt-Henn A, Horii A, et al. Diagnostic criteria for persistent postural-perceptual dizziness (PPPD): Consensus document of the Committee for the Classification of Vestibular Disorders of the Bárány Society. *J Vestib Res.* 2017;27:191–208.

Tirelli G, Nicastro L, Gatto A, Tofanelli M. Repeated canalith repositioning procedure in BPPV: Effects on recurrence and dizziness prevention. *Am J Otolaryngol.* 2017;38:38–43.

Vucovic, V, Plavec, D, Galinovic, L, et al. Prevalence of vertigo, dizziness, and migrainous vertigo in patients with migraine. *Headache.* 2007;47:1427–1435.

11 Cough Headache

Specialties: Neurology and Radiology

A 52-year-old man presents with a 2-week history of headache that developed during an upper respiratory illness. The headaches come on abruptly whenever he coughs or sneezes and are characterized by a sharp, stabbing sensation at the vertex and occiput lasting from 20 seconds to 2 minutes. He sometimes will have a dull headache linger for several hours afterward. He denies nausea, vomiting, photophobia, or phonophobia. His eyes do not water, and he does not have any cranial autonomic symptoms with his pain. At times, lifting heavy packages can trigger these attacks. He is exhausted, having been awakened multiple times each night by his upper respiratory illness–associated coughing fits and subsequent attacks of head pain. His medical examination is remarkable only for scattered rhonchi. The neurological examination is entirely normal. He has a history of migraine, and he states that these headaches are very different. He has been unable to treat these attacks because they are of such short duration.

What do you do now?

This case raises concern in that the headaches are of new onset and begin for the first time in a middle-aged man. In addition, these attacks of pain occur suddenly and follow maneuvers that increase intracranial pressure. Although the neurological examination is normal, the clinical history is suspicious for an intracranial lesion (see Chapters 14).

Headaches that occur with coughing, sneezing, straining, or exertion should prompt a search for lesions within the posterior fossa, craniocervical junction, or cerebrospinal fluid (CSF) pathways. Although cough and other exertional headaches are often linked together, they are distinct entities in the *International Classification of Headache Disorders*, third edition (ICHD-3). The diagnosis of the primary forms of these disorders can only be made after secondary forms have been excluded. Hence, neuroimaging is required.

Primary cough headache is uncommon, with a lifetime prevalence of approximately 1%. This condition more often affects men, typically older than age 40 years, and although often described as a severe headache of sudden onset, it is by definition benign. Within seconds of coughing, sneezing, straining, or other Valsalva maneuvers, an immediate headache is experienced. The headache usually subsides within 1 second to 30 minutes; however, some sufferers may continue to experience a dull ache for several hours afterward. The pain is usually described as sharp, stabbing, or splitting in nature; of moderate to severe intensity; and generally bilateral. Patients usually describe the pain as localized to the vertex, frontal, occipital, or temporal areas and without nausea, vomiting, or other neurological symptoms. The ICHD-3 diagnostic criteria for primary cough headache are listed in Box 11.1. Although the precise etiology is unknown, it may relate to a sudden increase in intracranial pressure with traction on pain-sensitive structures from a downward displacement of cerebellar tonsils.

When cough headache occurs in a younger patient, is of long duration, is strictly unilateral, or is associated with other features, we must have a high index of suspicion for a secondary cause, and a thorough workup must be done accordingly. Among other diagnoses, secondary cough headache has been described in Chiari malformation (see Chapter 6); brain tumors, both malignant and benign (meningioma/acoustic neuroma); cerebral aneurysm; and carotid or vertebrobasilar disease (see Chapter 5).

Primary exercise headache (PEH), previously referred to as primary exertional headache, not surprisingly, occurs with exertional effort, as may occur during physical exercise such as running or other forms of cardio. The headache is of sudden onset and often bilateral in location, but unlike cough headache, the pain is often pulsatile and of longer duration (5 minutes to 48 hours). The ICHD-3 criteria for primary exercise headache are listed in Box 11.2. It is worth noting that PEH can share features of migraine and is often experienced by individuals who also have migraine. Consequently, treatment options can overlap. PEH is an indomethacin-responsive headache, and in situations in which exercise is the only trigger, individuals may do just fine by taking indomethacin or propranolol prior to the activity. In other cases, if the headache attacks are frequent and the individual has comorbid migraine, it will be important to also address migraine with a preventive treatment.

As in cough headache, neuroimaging to rule out a posterior fossa or craniocervical junction abnormality should be undertaken in a patient presenting with new exercise headache, particularly when the headache is unilateral. In addition to unilaterality, secondary exercise headache often begins later in life, lasts longer (24 hours to weeks), and, in cases of subarachnoid hemorrhage, is associated with focal neurological features such as meningismus. Other secondary causes include Chiari malformation (see Chapter 6), subdural hematoma, neoplasm (primary and metastatic), venous sinus thrombosis, and platybasia. A "first-ever" presentation of exercise headache requires a workup with neuroimaging, including magnetic resonance imaging (MRI) of the brain, vascular imaging, and possibly also transcranial Doppler depending on the rest of the workup to rule out secondary causes, such as subarachnoid hemorrhage or arterial dissection (see Chapter 5).

Indomethacin is the treatment of choice in patients who frequently experience cough headache, and often the sustained-release formulation (75 mg once or twice daily) offers better clinical relief. In other instances, patients may do well with simply taking 25–50 mg prior to exercise. A positive response to indomethacin may be seen in secondary cases and is therefore not diagnostic of primary cough headache. Other agents that have been reported to offer benefit include naproxen, acetazolamide, propranolol, methysergide, dihydroergotamine, and topiramate. In a small case series, Raskin (1995) reported that lumbar puncture with removal of 40 cc of CSF provided prompt relief.

Although our patient meets all the clinical criteria for primary cough headache, he still needs further investigations to rule out intracranial pathology. MRI of the brain should be done. If the MRI results are normal, then a good treatment choice would be indomethacin 75 mg sustained-release daily along with a nonnarcotic cough suppressant. Education and reassurance are also important because patients need to be made aware that this is a self-limited benign problem.

KEY POINTS TO REMEMBER

- Cough headache is symptomatic in approximately 40% of cases and may be the result of lesions in the posterior fossa, craniocervical junction, or CSF pathways, so neuroimaging is required.
- Primary cough headache typically affects men older than age 40 years and is of short duration (1 second to 2 hours), bilateral, and unassociated with nausea or vomiting.
- Cough headache can be precipitated by coughing, sneezing, straining, or other Valsalva maneuvers.
- The treatment of choice is indomethacin, but in cases in which it is triggered solely by a cough and the situation is transient, a cough suppressant might be enough.

Further Reading

Halker RB, Vargas BB. Primary exertional headache: Updates in the literature. *Curr Pain Headache Rep.* 2013;17(6):337.

Newman LC, Grosberg BM, Dodick DW. Other primary headaches. In: Silberstein SD, Lipton RB, Dodick DW, eds. *Wolff's Headache and Other Head Pain.* 8th ed. New York, NY: Oxford University Press; 2008:431–447.

Pasqual J. Primary cough headache. *Curr Pain Headache Rep.* 2005;4:124–128.

Raskin NH. The cough headache syndrome: Treatment. *Neurology.* 1995;45:1784.

VanderPluym J. Indomethacin-responsive headaches. *Curr Neurol Neurosci Rep.* 2015;15(2):516.

Nummular Headache

A 54-year-old accountant describes pain "right here" (indicating an area approximately 1 inch in diameter in his right parietal region) for the past 3 months. He states that the pain is nearly constant, although it waxes and wanes, at times mild and not distracting. He thinks it can be triggered by cold air on his head or by scratching that area. He has noted some sharp "stabbing pains" in the same region. He thinks there has not been much nausea but admits to some "queasiness" when the pain persists at higher levels. The location of the pain never changes. He denies photosensitivity and phonosensitivity. He does not recall a recent head injury. Over-the-counter medications have not helped, and the triptan medication prescribed by his primary care provider has been ineffective as well. His neurological examination is normal, and although his painful area "doesn't feel right," it is not numb.

What do you do now?

Nummular ("coin-shaped") headache (NH) is characterized by generally continuous but usually not severe pain limited to a small area of the scalp. There can be sharp pains (lancinations) superimposed upon baseline aching pain. The parietal area seems to be the most common site. Sometimes the affected area is tender to the touch. In addition to pain, patients commonly experience decreased sensation in the area (or adjacent areas), dysesthesias (unpleasant sensation after non-noxious stimulus), and paresthesias. Neurological examination and neuroimaging are normal. There can be spontaneous periods of remission (see Box 12.1).

Diagnostic possibilities here include an intracranial mass; skull lesion; scalp infection or mass; and referred pain from a more distant head, face, or neck lesion. Less likely causes might include hemicrania continua (see Chapter 16), side-locked migraine, tension-type headache, giant cell arteritis (GCA; also known as temporal arteritis; see Chapter 4), and local neuralgias such as occipital and auriculotemporal neuralgia. Computed tomography or magnetic resonance imaging of the head and careful assessment of the scalp and head are generally sufficient to rule out secondary causes. Erythrocyte sedimentation rate (ESR) is worth checking to rule out GCA, but of note, an unusually high comorbidity with autoimmune disorders has been reported in NH, particularly Sjogren syndrome, which might also explain a high ESR.

Nummular headache is considered one of the "epicranias," which are postulated to be due to local scalp-generated neuropathic pain. In the case of NH, there is presumably dysfunction in a localized terminal branch of

---

BOX 12.1 **Diagnostic Criteria for Nummular Headache**

A. Continuous or intermittent head pain
B. Felt exclusively in an area of the scalp, with all of the following four characteristics:
  1. Sharply contoured
  2. Fixed in size and shape
  3. Round or elliptical
  4. 1–6 cm in diameter
C. Not better accounted for by another diagnosis

Adapted from the *International Classification of Headache Disorders*, third edition.

the trigeminal nerve. Pareja, who first described NH, reported a series of patients with NH who had trophic changes such as hair loss and skin depression in the area of the head pain, and suggested that these may herald the development of a complex regional pain syndrome (CRPS).

Treatment consists first of reassurance—that this is not a life-threatening disorder and that workup has revealed no cranial or intracranial lesion. Nonsteroidal anti-inflammatory medication seems to help patients with NH. Prophylactic medication helpful in other neuropathic pain conditions should also be considered. Gabapentin has been used successfully, and it is reasonable to consider other antiepileptic medications as well as tricyclic antidepressant medications. If there is suspicion of hemicrania continua, a trial of indomethacin is warranted, beginning at low dose and titrating upward to 75 mg three times daily for at least 1 week.

Alternatively, infiltration of the sensitive area with local anesthetic (LA) may be both diagnostic and therapeutic, with pain relief sometimes lasting much longer than the action of the LA. Agents that are useful include lidocaine 1% and bupivicaine 0.25%. Many employ a 1:1 mix of both of these and inject approximately 1 or 2 cc into the middle of the involved region, with the patient directing the location. The addition of corticosteroids along with LA is often done but probably adds no benefit and may lead to local alopecia. Local injection of botulinum toxin has been used for intractable cases. Radiofrequency nerve ablation has also been used successfully. Transcutaneous nerve stimulation over the involved area has helped some patients and may obviate the need for more invasive approaches. The possibility that NH may progress to a chronic form with features of CRPS might encourage early treatment.

KEY POINTS TO REMEMBER

- Focal head pain may be due to scalp, skull, or intracranial lesions, but when strictly localized to a coin-shaped area and associated with other sensory phenomena, it may represent NH.
- Nummular headache is thought to represent focal neuropathic pain and thus may respond to anti-neuralgia treatment.
- Infiltration of the area of pain with local anesthetic can be therapeutic as well as diagnostic.

Further Reading

Chen WH, Chen YT, Lin CS, Li TH, Lee LH, Chen CJ. A high prevalence of autoimmune indices and disorders in primary nummular headache. *J Neurol Sci.* 2012;320:127–130.

Dusitanond P, Young W. Botulinum toxin type A's efficacy in nummular headache. *Headache.* 2008;48:1379.

Headache Classification Committee of the International Headache Society. The *International Classification of Headache Disorders*, 3rd edition. *Cephalalgia.* 2018;38:1–211.

Martins IP, Abreu L. Nummular headache: Clinical features and treatment response in 24 new cases. *Cephalalgia Rep.* 2018;1:1–8.

13 Cervicogenic Headache

A 72-year-old woman is referred to your clinic by her primary care provider for further management of a new-onset headache. This began 5 months ago without clear precipitant. Pain is located in the right occiput with some radiation to right parietal regions. Pain is described as dull and "nagging." She notices the headache most while cooking or being active. Most over-the-counter analgesics she has used are ineffective, and the only thing that seems to alleviate pain is to lay down on her right side with her head propped up on a pillow in a specific way, which she demonstrates in your office. She had a computed tomography (CT) brain and basic lab work including erythrocyte sedimentation rate and C-reactive protein, which were all unremarkable. A previous clinician suspected she had cerebrospinal fluid (CSF) leak given improvement while lying down. She therefore had a CT myelogram, which was normal, and a subsequent nontargeted blood patch to no avail. She is frustrated because she has never had headaches before and is looking for "some relief." Her examination is normal with the exception of reduced range of motion of the neck and a positive Spurling sign.

What do you do now?

Although CSF leak was not an unreasonable consideration given the patient's headache was relieved while laying down, the key feature that permeates her history is that position and provocative maneuvers elicit the headache. The most likely diagnosis here is cervicogenic headache.

Cervicogenic headache is a secondary headache disorder in which pain is referred to the head from a source in the cervical spine. It can be challenging to diagnose because patients with headache and neck pain can often have overlapping diagnoses. Neck pain is not even an essential symptom for diagnosis. Neurological examination can be normal; however, a positive Spurling sign is often seen (Box 13.1). A Spurling test is a maneuver in which the examiner tilts the patient's head to the affected side while extending and applying downward pressure to the top of the patient's head. If this test reproduces the pain, this is considered a positive Spurling sign. The mechanism underlying many cases of cervicogenic headache involves convergence between upper cervical and trigeminal afferents in the spinal trigeminal nucleus. Structures capable of producing referred pain to the head are those innervated by the C1–C3 nerves. Pain from the C3–C4 joint can also be referred to the head. Structures innervated by lower cervical nerves have not been clearly shown to directly contribute to headaches.

BOX 13.1   **ICHD-3 Diagnostic Criteria for Cervicogenic Headache**

A. Any headache fulfilling criterion C
B. Clinical and/or imaging evidence of a disorder or lesion within the cervical spine or soft tissue of the neck, known to be able to cause headache
C. Evidence of causation demonstrated by at least two of the following:
   1. Headache has developed in temporal relation to the onset of the cervical disorder of the appearance of the lesion.
   2. Headache has significantly improved or resolved in parallel with improvement in or resolution of the cervical disorder or lesion.
   3. Cervical range of motion is reduced and headache is made significantly worse by provocative maneuvers.
   4. Headache is abolished following diagnostic blockade of a cervical structure or its nerve supply.
D. Not better accounted for by another ICHD-3 diagnosis

ICHD-3, *International Classification of Headache Disorders,* third edition. Adapted from ICHD-3.

Differential diagnosis of cervicogenic headache should be considered. The most crucial of these is dissection of the vertebral or internal carotid arteries, which can present with neck pain and headache. Lesions in the posterior cranial fossa should be eliminated as well. Meningitis of the upper cervical spine can be distinguished from cervicogenic headache by the presence of systemic illness and neck rigidity. Herpes zoster can produce pain in the occipital region during its prodromal phase; however, the eruption of vesicles distinguishes this disease from cervicogenic headache.

Diagnostic imaging of the cervical spine may be helpful although not necessary in diagnosing cervicogenic headache. If clinicians have the ability to undertake fluoroscopically guided diagnostic blocks, they can establish a cervical source of pain and validate the diagnoses. In addition, nerve blockade and subsequent pulsed radiofrequency treatment can be very beneficial for cervicogenic headache patients. For probable cervicogenic headache, or in circumstances in which diagnostic blocks are not an option, exercises with or without manual therapy seem to be the best option among conservative therapy. Pharmacological treatments are not well established; however, neuropathic medications, tricyclic antidepressants, as well muscle relaxants have been implored.

KEY POINTS TO REMEMBER

- Cervicogenic headache is a secondary headache disorder in which pain is referred to the head from a source in the cervical spine. Neck pain is not a necessary feature for diagnosis.
- The differential diagnosis includes posterior fossa lesions and dissections of either the vertebral artery or the internal carotid artery.
- Fluoroscopically guided diagnostic blocks can be both diagnostic and therapeutic.

Further Reading

Antonaci F, Ertugrul L. Headache and neck. *Cephalalgia*. 2021;4:438–442.

Antonaci F, Sjaastad O. Cervicogenic headache: A real headache. *Curr Neurol Neurosci Rep*. 2011;11:149–155.

Bogduk N, Govind J. Cervicogenic headache: An assessment of the evidence on clinical diagnosis, invasive tests, and treatment. *Lancet Neurol.* 2009;8:959–968.

Park MS, Hyuk JC, Yang JS, et al. Clinical efficacy of pulsed radiofrequency treatment targeting the mid-cervical medial branches for intractable cervicogenic headache. *Clin J Pain.* 2021;37:206–210.

14 Thunderclap Headache

A 31-year-old woman developed a new headache
3 weeks ago. She was swimming laps in her local
community pool when she experienced a sudden
and severe holocephalic headache. She states she
was unable to move for several minutes due to the
pain. However, the pain eventually "let up," and she
was able to get out of the water and go home and
rest, with resolution of the pain. Because she quickly
recovered, she thought she may have kinked her neck
and decided not to seek treatment. However, this
headache recurred 3 days later when she was at the
grocery store. The pain was again sudden, severe, and
per patient "brought me to my knees." This time, she
also felt her vision was blurry and that her right side
felt slightly weak compared to the left. She therefore
decided to go to the local emergency department.
She denies nausea, vomiting, photophobia, and
phonophobia. Neurological examination is entirely
normal. Past medical history is significant only for
mild anxiety, for which she recently started a selective
serotonin reuptake inhibitor (SSRI) with her primary
care physician. Head magnetic resonance imaging
(MRI) and lumbar puncture were negative.

What do you do now?

This case is worrisome for several reasons. First, this is a new headache in a patient who has not had headaches in the past—although not unheard of and certainly age 31 years is a possible time for onset of a number of primary headaches. Second, there are reported accompanying transient neurological signs of decreased visual acuity and focal weakness. Last, the sudden and severe onset is pathognomonic for thunderclap headache, a worrisome and potential sentinel headache that should never be overlooked.

In this case, the normal MRI essentially excludes mass lesions. Recurrent intracerebral hemorrhages or subarachnoid bleeding is probably also ruled out by the normal MRI and clear cerebrospinal fluid (CSF). However, there is the specter of symptomatic unruptured aneurysms or aneurysmal "sentinel" bleeding, both of which may have been missed. Migraine without nausea and phono-/photophobia is distinctly unlikely, and true weakness as an aura symptom (hemiplegic migraine) is quite rare.

This patient's syndrome is, in fact, most typical of the so-called reversible cerebral vasoconstriction syndromes (RCVS). These represent a group of disorders characterized by recurring thunderclap headaches and reversible vasoconstriction of cerebral arteries, leading to neurological signs and symptoms of various degrees, presenting over days to weeks. There are a number of synonyms for the general syndrome, including Call–Fleming syndrome, benign angiopathy of the central nervous system (CNS), and thunderclap headache with reversible vasospasm. Probably, RCVS includes a number of cases of drug-induced cerebral arteritis. The etiology of RCVS is not clear, but it can occur coincidently with certain medication or drug use, such as initiation of SSRIs (as seen in this case). Pregnancy and postpartum period have been reported as a vulnerable time period for RCVS as well. It is differentiated from primary angiitis of the CNS by its normal CSF. It is diagnosed by reversible segmental cerebral arterial constriction on angiography.

Differential diagnosis for thunderclap headache, however, also includes cervical artery dissection, cerebral venous sinus thrombosis, cerebral hemorrhage (lobar and cerebellar), cerebral vasculitis and spontaneous intracranial hypotension, pituitary apoplexy, and of course the most notable cause of thunderclap headache, subarachnoid hemorrhage (SAH) (Box 14.1).

Given the potentially serious outcome of its possible underlying causes, thunderclap headache should always be considered a medical emergency.

> **BOX 14.1 Potential Causes of Thunderclap Headache**
>
> Subarachnoid hemorrhage
> Intracranial hemorrhage (lobar or cerebellar)
> Cerebral venous thrombosis
> Cerebral vasculitis
> Cervical artery dissection
> Spontaneous intracranial hypotension
> Pituitary apoplexy
> Acute hypertensive crises
> Reversible cerebral vasoconstrictive syndrome
> Third ventricle colloid cyst
> Intracranial infection
> Primary thunderclap headache
> Primary cough, sexual, and exertional headache

The initial diagnostic assessment must be focused on first ruling out SAH. Noncontrast CT of the brain, the first test in this assessment, is highly sensitive and specific for the diagnosis of SAH when done in close temporal relationship to the onset of symptoms. During the first 12 hours after the onset of headache is ideal. Given that the sensitivity of CT is not perfect, CSF should be obtained in patients who present with thunderclap headache and who have normal or nondiagnostic CT scans. If CT of the brain and CSF analysis are unremarkable, an MRI should be done; in most cases, this should also include some form of head and neck vessel imaging, including MR angiography or CT angiography. Conventional angiography is not a necessary component in the assessment of patients with thunderclap headache. It is also a procedure that is not risk-free. However, it may be necessary in select cases when clinical suspicion for RCVS remains high despite normal or nondiagnostic testing.

Treatment of thunderclap headache is dependent on underlying etiology. If RCVS is diagnosed as in this patient, indicated treatment is thought to include the calcium channel blockers nimodipine or verapamil and possibly corticosteroids. If no underlying etiology is identified, a diagnosis of either primary thunderclap headache or primary cough, exertional, or sexual headache should be considered. Indomethacin 25–50 mg either daily or prior to provoking activity is the treatment of choice for these primary thunderclap headaches.

KEY POINTS TO REMEMBER

- Thunderclap headache is an excruciating headache that reaches maximal intensity in less than 1 minute.
- Thunderclap headache should always be considered a medical emergency. The initial diagnostic assessment must be focused on first ruling out SAH with a noncontrast CT of the brain and lumbar puncture. Further diagnostic testing, including MRI brain with vascular imaging, may be necessary.
- Diagnosis of primary thunderclap headache should only be made after all other possible etiologies have been excluded.

Further Reading

Calabrese LH, Dodick DW, Schwedt TJ, Singhal AB. Narrative review: Reversible cerebral vasoconstriction syndromes. *Ann Intern Med.* 2007;146:34–44.

Koppin H, van Sonderen A, et al. Thunderclap headache. In: Ferrari A, Charles A, eds. *Oxford Textbook of Headache Syndromes.* New York, NY: Oxford University Press; 2020:307–313.

Schwedt T, Dodick D, Matharu M. Thunderclap headache. *Lancet Neurol.* 2006;5:621–631.

Yang CW, Fuh JL. Thunderclap headache: An update. *Expert Rev Neurotherapeut.* 2018;18 (12):915–924.

Treatment Questions

15　Medication Overuse

Specialties: Neurology, Primary Care, and Communication Skills

A 42-year-old woman with daily headache is in your office for the first time. She has a history consistent with migraine that dates back to age 20 years, and during the past 3 years, her headaches have been gradually worsening so that she now experiences daily headache without moments of pain freedom. She brings an extensive list of medications she has already tried and explains that nothing has helped; the only medication that allows her to function is sumatriptan 100 mg, which she takes once daily. She adds that several times in the past, she was able to stop all acute medications for approximately 1 month but did not experience any headache change. Two previous hospitalizations for treatment with intravenous dihydroergotamine resulted in relief of headache pain only during the hospitalizations; her pain returned to the prehospitalization level within 3 days of discharge. Prior workup was normal. Current medical and neurological exams are normal. Although you counsel her about acute medication limits, she asks, "Why do I need to stop taking sumatriptan daily? My headaches are exactly the same whether I take it or not, but at least I have some relief when I can treat them."

What do you do now?

This is an uncommon but not a rare occurrence in headache subspecialty practices that poses a conundrum. In essence, we need to ask ourselves why treatment is not working. And if we determine that everything appropriate was done, how can we guarantee that there will not be dose escalation and the headache will not continue to worsen if the patient continues to use even limited amounts of the medication? Furthermore, what are the potential long-term consequences of daily analgesic use?

There can be many reasons why a treatment is not effective. Often, the headache diagnosis is wrong, whereas other times the diagnosis is incomplete. Migraine may be misdiagnosed as sinus or tension-type headache; paroxysmal hemicrania may be mistaken for cluster. A more worrisome scenario occurs when a secondary headache disorder is misidentified as a primary headache. Sometimes, the patient suffers from more than one headache diagnosis. Treating one headache diagnosis while ignoring the other(s) will lead to an incomplete treatment response.

Other common reasons for treatment failure include inappropriate or subtherapeutic pharmacotherapy. Although the patient usually states that they have been prescribed all available medications, it is important to review the maximum dosage reached, the duration of treatment, and the actual response to the therapy. Ensure that the medication was begun at a low dose, gradually increased, and continued for a proper therapeutic trial. Simply accepting a list of names of medications tried is not sufficient.

Frequently, patients discontinue a medication before it can be of benefit. In general, a trial of 4–6 weeks at a target dose is needed to evaluate efficacy. Discuss reasons for medication discontinuation, because treatment is often stopped inappropriately. Medication side effects may be misinterpreted as allergic reactions, or a self-limited reaction (paresthesias, sedation, etc.) is misperceived as too disabling or potentially permanent.

Very commonly, treatment failure is the result of a coexistent precipitating or exacerbating factor that has been overlooked. Issues to be explored include diet (caffeine overuse or withdrawal, artificial sweeteners, and missed or irregular mealtimes), sleep patterns, stress, and hormonal status. Comorbid medical disorders such as anxiety, depression, cardiac disease, or pulmonary disease, or even the medications used to treat these conditions, may worsen the headaches or interfere with the treatment. Most important, the clinician must search for medication overuse. The frequent use (daily or near daily) of acute medications, including over-the-counter analgesics, is the most common cause of treatment refractoriness yet is often not addressed and sometimes not recognized. These medications can induce "rebound" headache, now termed medication overuse headache (MOH) by the third edition of the *International Classification of Headache Disorders*, and limit the effectiveness of the migraine preventives.

The frequency of analgesic use required to produce MOH is not clear, and there is probably a fair amount of individual variation among patients. However, an average minimum frequency is approximately 2 or 3 days per week. If patients keep their use of all analgesics and other acute medication to a total of less than 2 days per week, most will not fall into the MOH pattern. And use of multiple agents on different days does not exempt patients from the risk—that is, they need to avoid *all* acute medications 5 days per week. Medication overuse also, of course, may lead to psychological dependence, medication tolerance, and withdrawal syndromes.

Most patients with MOH can be treated on an outpatient basis. Depending on the medication, patients are either slowly weaned (for butalbital, narcotics, and caffeine-containing products) or can be abruptly discontinued (simple analgesics, ergots, and triptans) while preventive medications are initiated. "Bridging therapies" should be employed as a stopgap measure to treat breakthrough pain. These transitional therapies, such as long-acting nonsteroidal anti-inflammatory drugs (NSAIDs), may be used to prevent acute pain flare-ups that can occur as an overused acute analgesic is being stopped and a preventive treatment is started. Occasionally, a tapering course of prednisone or other steroid, such as a Medrol dose pak or dexamethasone, over 1 week or so is instituted to break the pain cycle as the preventive agents are started. Severe attacks may be treated with triptans or dihydroergotamine nasal spray, but the patient must be limited to no more than two treatments weekly. If the patient is overusing caffeine-containing medications, care must be taken to slowly wean the patient from all sources of caffeine.

If the patient is overusing butalbital-containing medications in small quantities (one to five tablets daily), a reasonable approach would be to decrease the intake by one tablet per day per week. In patients whose intake is greater than five tablets daily, switching the short-acting butalbital to longer acting phenobarbital is a better option. Using this strategy, 30 mg of phenobarbital is substituted for every 100 mg of butalbital (Fiorinal and Esgic contain 50 mg per tablet) and tapered by 15–30 mg daily. Opioids should be tapered by 10–15% every week. Clonidine 1 mg bid–tid is useful for reducing withdrawal symptoms. It is important to educate patients that even though pain medications, including opioids, might be used to treat other pain conditions, in an individual with migraine, they still carry the risk of contributing to MOH and chronification of migraine if used more than 2 days per week.

While the overused analgesic is being stopped and a new acute medication started, this is also a good time to ensure preventive therapy is being maximized and consider nonpharmacological options, such as biofeedback, cognitive–behavioral therapy (CBT), or even a noninvasive neuromodulation device. A multifactorial approach to pain management can be very helpful.

These issues related to treatment and acute medication use should be addressed and then re-explored over the course of follow-up visits. By reviewing old records and interviewing the patient (it is often very useful to reinterview the patient as if it was the initial consultation), past inadequacies may be brought into focus and new options discovered. For truly refractory patients, a second opinion can uncover clues previously overlooked.

On a first visit, it is prudent to rethink or even redo the diagnostic workup. Were all options attempted? Were dosages correct and therapeutic trials sufficiently long? Were medications used in combination and behavioral therapies employed? Were nerve blocks or other interventional techniques attempted? Usually, the savvy clinician can find treatment options that were not utilized. It might also be worthwhile to attempt an inpatient admission to a center in which a longer stay and a more aggressive treatment approach, utilizing intravenous dihydroergotamine as well as additional intravenous medications and other therapies, could be attempted.

A more difficult situation arises when the patient in question is an established one—a patient the clinician knows well and for whom all reasons for treatment unresponsiveness have been eliminated. This patient has tried medications in combination, biobehavioral and invasive therapies, and appropriate, long-duration, aggressive inpatient treatment. Despite this appropriate care and in the setting of long periods (months) of analgesic washout, they continue to suffer from ongoing, disabling headaches. Do you allow them to use daily analgesics and, if so, which ones, as they differ in their potential for toxicity, abuse, and dependence? If you have access to a Comprehensive Pain Rehabilitation Program, in which an intensive multimodal approach to pain management is used, these patients often do quite well with a referral.

It is the rare patient who can use daily analgesics without the subsequent need for dose escalation, but those patients do exist. In this case, we could consider allowing the patient to continue if the daily medication was a simple analgesic or NSAID. In these circumstances, the clinician must explain the risks and benefits of prolonged usage (cardiac, nephrotoxic, gastrointestinal, etc.), documenting this in the patient's chart with a notation that the patient is aware of the potential consequences and believes the benefits outweigh the risks. These patients need to be very closely monitored with frequent office visits and laboratory testing. On the other hand, if the patient insists on continuing a narcotic medication, an ergotamine preparation, or a triptan, many headache specialists would be significantly more reticent and more than likely prohibit it.

The evidence does not support the use of chronic opioid therapy for most patients with chronic daily headache. A 5-year study of 300 patients with intractable headaches treated with long-acting opioids found that only 20% of patients were significantly improved and 40% demonstrated some aspects of noncompliance (Saper and Lake 2006) The authors recommended that long-term opioid therapy should be reserved for only those patients who have failed all reasonable treatment options, including hospitalization and detoxification, and who are without axis I psychiatric or personality disorders. There has also been a more recent retrospective cohort study (Shao et al. 2021) demonstrating that emergency department utilization of opioids to treat migraine led to more frequent health resource utilization, highlighting the importance of treating migraine appropriately, even in the emergency department setting.

There is good evidence for the use of topiramate in patients with chronic migraine and MOH; consequently, fully understanding previous treatment trials with topiramate and carefully outlining expectations including benign/transient and serious side effects are important because it might be worth retrying topiramate. Combination prevention therapies can also be helpful—for example, a patient could be started on both topiramate and onabotulinumtoxinA. When combining preventive treatments, it makes sense to choose medications from different classes that may have different mechanisms of action.

Because MOH is a secondary headache and by definition associated with people who have an underlying primary headache diagnosis such as migraine, a quality improvement update was jointly published in 2020 by the American Headache Society and the American Academy of Neurology in the journals *Headache* and *Neurology* to maximize dissemination provide guidance on outpatient headache management, including management of MOH. Clinicians are recommended to consider medication overuse in the context of the underlying primary headache disorder and include management of MOH as one part of their overall treatment plan as they address the primary headache diagnosis, rather than approaching the situation as if the patient has two different concurrent headache diagnoses. The work group members did this with intention: There was concern that when MOH was treated as a separate entity from the concurrent primary headache disorder, it was given disproportionate attention and there was underutilization of preventive medications.

We are in the midst of a paradigm shift in migraine management. The U.S. Food and Drug Administration (FDA) approval of calcitonin gene-related peptide (CGRP) monoclonal antibodies for migraine prevention has opened up a new class of drugs to patients who otherwise have tried so many other treatments that we have to offer. These drugs can be effective even in patients who have not found other preventives to help and also when MOH is a concern. The new noninvasive neuromodulation devices, which are FDA cleared for acute and preventive therapy, can also be very helpful when MOH might be playing a role. Patients who have been using daily acute analgesics often feel reassured if they have an acute treatment option they can use without restrictions, and noninvasive neuromodulation devices can be used daily without worry of MOH. CGRP small molecule antagonists (referred to as "gepants") are also now available for the acute treatment of migraine, and the data support that they do not contribute to MOH. In fact, with this finding and additional trial data from preventive studies, rimegepant has become the first class of migraine drug treatment to be approved for both acute and preventive therapy.

In patients who believe they have "tried everything," consider a multimodal approach: a preventive treatment for migraine, an acute treatment limited to no more than 2 days per week, and possibly a noninvasive neuromodulation device or other nonpharmacologic therapies such as biofeedback or CBT.

KEY POINTS TO REMEMBER

- Refractory daily headache is usually the result of misdiagnosis, inappropriate or inadequate pharmacotherapy, or failure to identify and treat coexisting exacerbating factors.
- Refractory daily headache commonly occurs in the setting of medication overuse.
- Refractory daily headache often requires inpatient hospitalization for detoxification and treatment.
- Chronic opioid therapy has a poor success rate and is often associated with noncompliance (dose violations, lost prescriptions, and multiple prescribers). It is generally not recommended for the long-term treatment of migraine and other primary headache disorders.
- Updated quality improvement measures recommend treating medication overuse as part of the primary headache disorder with which it is associated rather than considering MOH as a distinct and separate entity. This will allow a greater likelihood that preventive treatments will be maximized, and disproportionate attention will not be given solely to MOH.
- Gepants are the first class of acute migraine medication not associated with the development of MOH.
- A multimodal approach is generally best in patients with refractory daily headache: (1) Stop overused acute analgesics; (2) address comorbid conditions that might be impacting headache; (3) start a preventive treatment; (4) provide an acute treatment with limitations of no more than 2 days per week; and (5) add a nonpharmacological therapy, such as a noninvasive neuromodulation device, biofeedback, or CBT.

Further Reading

American Headache Society. The American Headache Society position statement on integrating new migraine treatments into clinical practice. *Headache*. 2019;59(1):1-18. doi:10.1111/head.13456

Croop R, Lipton RB, Kudrow D, et al. Oral rimegepant for preventive treatment of migraine: A phase 2/3, randomised, double-blind, placebo-controlled trial. *Lancet*. 2021;397:51-60. doi:10.1016/S0140-6736(20)32544-7

Diener HC, Bussone G, Van Oene JC, Lahaye M, Schwalen S, Goadsby PJ; TOPMAT-MIG-201(TOP-CHROME) Study Group. Topiramate reduces headache days in chronic migraine: A randomized, double-blind, placebo-controlled study. *Cephalalgia*. 2007;27(7):814–823.

Halker Singh RB, Ailani J, Robbins MS. Neuromodulation for the acute and preventive therapy of migraine and cluster headache. *Headache*. 2019;59(Suppl. 2):33–49. doi:10.1111/head.13586

Lipton RB, Silberstein SD, Saper J, Goadsby PJ. Why headache treatment fails. *Neurology*. 2003;60:1064–1070.

Navratilova E, Behravesh S, Oyarzo J, Dodick DW, Banerjee P, Porreca F. Ubrogepant does not induce latent sensitization in a preclinical model of medication overuse headache. *Cephalalgia*. 2020;40(9):892-902. doi:10.1177/0333102420938652

Robbins MS, Victorio MC, Bailey M, et al. Quality improvement in neurology: Headache Quality Measurement Set. *Neurology*. 2020;95(19):866–873. doi:10.1212/WNL.0000000000010634

Robbins MS, Victorio MCC, Bailey M, et al. Quality improvement in neurology: Headache Quality Measurement Set. *Headache*. 2021;61(1):219-226. doi:10.1111/head.13988

Saper JR, Lake AE. Sustained opioid therapy should rarely be administered to headache patients: Clinical observations, literature review, and proposed guidelines. *Headache Currents*. 2006;3:67–70.

Shao Q, Rascati KL, Lawson KA, Wilson JP, Shah S, Garrett JS. Impact of emergency department opioid use on future health resource utilization among patients with migraine. *Headache*. 2021;61(2):287–299. doi:10.1111/head.14071

Sheftell FD, Rapoport AM, Tepper SJ, Bigal ME. Naratriptan in the preventive treatment of refractory transformed migraine: A prospective pilot study. *Headache*. 2005;45:1400–1406.

VanderPluym JH. Once too many: Impact of emergency department opioid use on future health resource utilization among patients with migraine. *Headache*. 2021;61(2):229–230. doi:10.1111/head.14070.

16 Hemicrania Continua

Specialty: Neurology

A 42-year-old woman with a 7-year history of daily headaches presents for an initial consultation. Her headache is present every waking moment and just fluctuates in intensity, and it has been this way for as long as she can remember. She reports that her pain is throbbing, moderate to severe, and accompanied by nausea and some light and sound sensitivity. Throughout the years, she has tried many different migraine preventive medications, as well as nonsteroidal anti-inflammatory drugs (NSAIDs) and a few different triptans including rizatriptan and naratriptan, without benefit. Upon further questioning, she reveals that her pain is strictly side-locked to the right: "Doc, if you just cut my head down the middle and remove the right side, I'd be ok!" She adds that when the pain is most severe, the headache is associated with tearing of the right eye and congestion of the right nostril. Her neurological examination is normal, as are the three recent head magnetic resonance images that she brought to the visit. She is currently taking an H_2-blocker because her recent endoscopy revealed multiple gastric erosions from overuse of aspirin.

What do you do now?

This patient has very bad luck. She is suffering from hemicrania continua (HC), a disabling headache condition, and multiple gastric erosions, which prohibits prescribing the treatment of choice. HC is an underrecognized, primary headache disorder and a common cause of refractory, unilateral, chronic daily headache. The disorder demonstrates a marked female preponderance, with a female-to-male ratio of approximately 2:1. The age at onset ranges from 11 to 58 years. HC is often an undiagnosed condition given its clinical overlap with migraine, and patients often spend years suffering before it is identified and appropriately treated. A hallmark of HC, which differentiates it from migraine, is its immediate and complete response to indomethacin. In migraine, patients may experience some temporary pain reduction with indomethacin given that it is an NSAID, whereas with HC, the pain should be completely resolved within a few days of starting treatment.

Clinically, HC is characterized by a unilateral, continuous headache of mild to moderate intensity. Patients usually describe this baseline discomfort as dull, aching, or pressing, and it is not associated with other symptoms. The pain is maximal in the ocular, temporal, and maxillary regions. Superimposed upon this background discomfort, exacerbations of more severe pain, lasting 20 minutes to several days, are experienced by the majority of people with HC. Although significantly more intense than the baseline pain, these painful exacerbations never reach the level experienced by those who have cluster headache. During these flare-ups, one or more autonomic symptoms (ptosis, conjunctival injection, lacrimation, and nasal congestion) occur ipsilateral to the pain. These exacerbations may occur at any time and frequently awaken the patient from sleep. Migrainous symptoms, such as nausea, vomiting, photophobia, and phonophobia, may also accompany the exacerbations of pain. Many patients report primary stabbing headaches (stabs and jabs) and a feeling of sand or an eyelash in the affected eye (foreign body sensation). Most patients experience strictly unilateral headaches without side shift, although there have been three patients described in whom attacks alternated sides, and another three bilateral cases have also been reported.

Two temporal profiles of HC exist: an episodic form, with distinct headache phases separated by pain-free remissions, and a chronic form, in which headaches persist without remissions.

Often, clinicians who are unfamiliar with HC will misdiagnose the disorder. If the physician focuses on the ipsilateral autonomic features that accompany the painful exacerbations, the disorder may be incorrectly diagnosed as cluster headache. Similarly, by focusing on the associated photophobia, phonophobia, nausea, and vomiting that may occur during exacerbations, HC may be misdiagnosed as migraine. It is distinguished from cluster and migraine by the presence of a continuous baseline headache of mild to moderate severity; neither the ipsilateral autonomic features of cluster nor the associated phenomena typically reported with migraine accompany this baseline pain.

Secondary mimics of HC have been reported to occur in association with a mesenchymal tumor involving the sphenoid bone, clinoid process, and skull base, as well as with pituitary lesions.

Indomethacin is the treatment of choice for HC, and response to therapy with indomethacin is required by the *International Classification of Headache Disorders*, third edition (ICHD-3), among the criteria for establishing the diagnosis. Therapy is usually initiated at a dose of 25 mg tid and increased to 50 mg tid in 1 week if there is no response or only partial benefit. Headache resolution is usually prompt, occurring within 1 or 2 days after the effective dosage is reached, although response may take as long as 2 weeks. Maintenance with doses ranging from 25 to 100 mg usually suffices; however, at times doses as high as 300 mg daily may be required.

Dosage adjustments are occasionally necessary to treat the clinical fluctuations that are sometimes seen with HC. Nighttime dosing with sustained-release indomethacin often prevents nocturnal exacerbations. During the active headache cycle, patients report that skipping or even delaying doses of indomethacin may result in the prompt reemergence of symptoms. The gastrointestinal side effects of indomethacin can be mitigated with antacids, misoprostol, or histamine H_2 receptor antagonists. These agents should always be considered for patients requiring long-term therapy. Although ICHD-3 requires indomethacin responsiveness as a diagnostic criterion, other agents have been reported to induce a partial response. These include naproxen, paracetamol, paracetamol with caffeine, ibuprofen, piroxicam, celecoxib, melatonin, gabapentin, and topiramate.

Because our patient has multiple gastric erosions, the use of indomethacin or other NSAIDs is contraindicated. In her case and for other patients in whom these agents are ineffective or prohibited, treatment with melatonin, gabapentin, or topiramate could be tried. Melatonin should be initiated at a dose of 3 mg at bedtime and can be increased by 3 mg every 3–5 nights, up to a maximum dosage of 24 mg nightly. Both topiramate and gabapentin are dosed in HC as they are in the treatment of migraine. Some patients find cranial nerve blocks to be helpful, and there is anecdotal evidence for pregabalin, amitriptyline, and duloxetine. With the advent of the new anti-calcitonin gene-related peptide drugs, it will be interesting to see if these will be helpful for HC, particularly given the clinical phenotypic overlap with migraine. After her erosions heal and if these other treatments are not effective, an indomethacin trial and one or more of the gastric protective agents may be employed, with the permission and supervision of her gastroenterologist. In this case, the patient would also need monitoring with periodic checks of her hemoglobin/hematocrit as well as her renal functioning because she would likely be on indomethacin long-term if it is beneficial.

KEY POINTS TO REMEMBER

- Hemicrania continua is an underrecognized cause of chronic daily headache.
- Hemicrania continua is characterized by a continuous, unilateral headache of mild to moderate severity.
- Superimposed exacerbations of pain, lasting minutes to days, occur and are associated with one or more ipsilateral autonomic features typical of cluster headache.
- Exacerbations may also be associated with migrainous features of nausea, vomiting, photophobia, and phonophobia.
- Many patients report stabbing "ice pick"-like headaches or a foreign body sensation in the ipsilateral eye.
- Indomethacin is the treatment of choice.
- Melatonin, gabapentin, and topiramate may relieve the pain and should be tried in patients who are intolerant of or prohibited from taking indomethacin.

Further Reading

Brighina F, Palermo A, Cosentino G, Fierro B. Prophylaxis of hemicrania continua: Two new cases effectively treated with topiramate. *Headache.* 2007;47:441–443.

Hryvenko I, Cervantes-Chavarría AR, Law AS, Nixdorf DR. Hemicrania continua: Case series presenting in an orofacial pain clinic. *Cephalalgia.* 2018;38(13):1950–1959. doi:10.1177/0333102418764895

Mehta A, Chilakamarri P, Zubair A, Kuruvilla DE. Hemicrania continua: A clinical perspective on diagnosis and management. *Curr Neurol Neurosci Rep.* 2018;18(2):95.

Peres MFP, Silberstein SD, Nahmias S, et al. Hemicrania continua is not that rare. *Neurology.* 2001;57:948–951.

Rozen TD. Melatonin responsive hemicrania continua. *Headache.* 2006;46:1203–1209.

Summ O, Andreou AP, Akerman S, Holland PR, Hoffmann J, Goadsby PJ. Differential actions of indomethacin: Clinical relevance in headache. *Pain.* 2021;162(2):591–599. doi:10.1097/j.pain.0000000000002032

17 Trigeminal Neuralgia

A 74-year-old man diagnosed with "tic douloureux" describes lancinating and aching pain in his right upper teeth and below his right eye for the past 8 months. Pain is sometimes brought on by chewing, blowing his nose (or at times even breathing through his nose), and brushing his teeth. There is occasional radiation of pain to the ear and throat ipsilaterally. He initially responded to carbamazepine, but this, despite dose escalation, has lost effectiveness. Neither baclofen nor pregabalin has been helpful. The pain is interfering with sleep, and while you are interviewing him, he seems to experience sudden stabs of pain. Past medical history is remarkable for stable coronary artery disease and sleep apnea. He is unaware of any instigating or associated events such as head trauma, facial rash, or dental work prior to the onset of pain.

What do you do now?

Syndromes of pain in the distribution of the trigeminal nerve can be caused by mechanical compression or irritation of the trigeminal nerve; by an inflammatory, neoplastic, or infectious condition in the face or cranium; or in many cases by idiopathic mechanisms. When some or all of the pain is lancinating, the term trigeminal neuralgia (TN) is applied. When the pain is more aching or burning and constant in character, it is generally considered more of a "painful trigeminal neuropathy," and sensation loss in one or more divisions of the trigeminal nerve is often noted on examination. But the boundaries are not distinct in some patients who display features of both broad categories. And some secondary processes can lead to either a neuralgic or a painful neuropathic presentation.

The current classification of TN subdivides conditions into (1) primary TN, either classical (due to proven neurovascular contact between the trigeminal nerve and a local artery) or idiopathic (no evidence of neurovascular contact); and (2) secondary TN caused by local pathology affecting the trigeminal nerve (other than neurovascular contact), such as masses, a multiple sclerosis lesion, or trauma (including trauma sustained during oral or facial procedures) (Box 17.1). TN is relatively rare, affecting approximately 0.1% of people.

Trigeminal neuralgia is more common in the elderly. It tends to involve the second and/or third divisions of the trigeminal nerve predominantly.

BOX 17.1 **Classification of Trigeminal Nerve Pain Syndromes**

Primary TN (generally intermittent lancinating pain, although it may be constant)
    Classical (proven neurovascular contact)
    Idiopathic (no evidence of neurovascular contact)
Secondary TN caused by local pathology affecting the trigeminal nerve
Painful trigeminal neuropathy
    Zoster infection
    Masses
    Cavernous sinus pathology
    Trauma
    Dental procedures or local anesthesia

TN, trigeminal neuralgia.

Typically, the pain is brief and "knife-like" (i.e., lancinating), severe, and often triggered by some sensory stimulus in a "trigger zone" that can be in the territory of the pain or nearby. There is often a "refractory period" during which pain will not occur even if triggered. Triggers include chewing, swallowing, washing the face, shaving, brushing the teeth, or even a breeze on the face. The pain sometimes causes a sudden facial muscle spasm that can look like a facial tic (hence the name tic douloureux). Sometimes the pain persists between attacks. Examination is generally normal.

Some cases of secondary TN are due to compression or irritation of the trigeminal nerve by a tumor, meningeal infectious process, demyelinating lesion around the trigeminal root entry zone, or zoster infection of the nerve. When these secondary causes are ruled out, compression of the trigeminal nerve by an arterial loop has been postulated as the most likely cause, and numerous examples of this have been seen in neuroimaging and in the operating room. Arteries most often found in the vicinity are the superior cerebellar artery and the anterior and posterior inferior cerebellar arteries. Some cases of TN seem to overlap with the syndrome of glossopharyngeal neuralgia (GN), described as similar lancinations but in the throat, posterior tongue, and ear, and typically triggered by swallowing. GN also occurs in older age groups, and it is more likely than TN to be due to a mass lesion somewhere along the length of the glossopharyngeal or vagus nerves.

The differential diagnosis of TN includes dental disease, sinus disease, cluster headache, giant cell arteritis, SUNCT/SUNA syndrome (short-lasting neuralgiform headaches with autonomic features), post-herpetic neuralgia, and idiopathic stabbing headache ("jabs and jolts"). Some cases seem to follow a dental procedure, with the supposition that some injury to a branch of the trigeminal was sustained. Skin rash may be fleeting or inapparent in some cases of zoster, which makes this etiology elusive. High-resolution magnetic resonance imaging (MRI), should be performed because secondary TN and TN mimics may not be ruled out clinically. Also, if arterial indentation of the trigeminal nerve is seen on imaging, microvascular decompression is more likely to be beneficial.

Our case seems to share features of both TN and GN (the two can coexist in approximately 10% of cases), so a search for secondary causes should be undertaken, with MRI of the head prior to and following gadolinium infusion to rule out brainstem or skull base mass lesions. If this is normal, a lumbar puncture might be considered to rule out an infectious or inflammatory etiology such as nonbacterial meningitis, sarcoidosis, Lyme disease, etc. Erythrocyte sedimentation rate should be done, as should a thorough dental evaluation (Box 17.2 provides a list of the common secondary causes of TN).

When workup fails to reveal a secondary cause of TN, medical therapy should be instituted. For prophylaxis of TN, a number of medications have proven useful, particularly carbamazepine (200–1200 mg daily) and oxcarbazepine (300–1800 mg daily). Gabapentin, lamotrigine, pregabalin, baclofen, and phenytoin may be used either alone or as adjunct therapy. Botulinum toxin type A has met with success in a number of cases, but the dosage and location of injections have varied highly in different reports, so recommending it can be challenging. Other medications can be helpful if these approaches fail (Table 17.1). Combining medications from different categories helps some patients for whom monotherapy failed. Tolerability and medication interactions limit the use of all of these options, particularly in the elderly, but careful dosage adjustment may allow titration to effective doses, even when two or three medications are used simultaneously. Carbamazepine, gabapentin, oxcarbazepine, and phenytoin are available in long-acting versions, which improves compliance and possibly tolerability. Medications that work well for TN tend to also work for GN.

For acute exacerbations of pain, benzodiazepines such as lorazepam or diazepam can help orally, but intravenous lorazepam is particularly useful in the emergency room setting for very severe pain. Intravenous infusions of fosphenytoin or lidocaine can also be used. (Intravenous phenytoin carries a risk of severe tissue damage if it extravasates, so it is to be avoided.)

TABLE 17.1 Pharmacologic Treatment of Trigeminal Neuralgia

Medication	Typical Effective Dosage
Carbamazepine (Tegretol®)	100–800 mg daily as tid po regimen
Oxcarbazepine (Trileptal®)	300–1800 mg daily as tid po regimen
Gabapentin (Neurontin®)	300–3600 mg daily as tid po regimen
Pregabalin (Lyrica®)	100–200 mg po tid
Lamotrigine (Lamictal®)	200–400 mg daily as tid po regimen
Phenytoin (Dilantin®)	100 mg po tid
Baclofen	10–60 mg daily as tid po regimen
Amitriptyline	10–150 mg po qhs
Nortriptyline	10–75 mg po qhs
Clonazepam (Klonipin®)	0.5–1 mg tid

Regarding surgical treatment of trigeminal neuralgia, there are three general approaches:

1. Microvascular decompression, involving suboccipital craniotomy under general anesthesia and physical transposition of arterial structures away from the trigeminal nerve ("Janetta"-type procedures)
2. "Gamma knife" radiosurgery to lesion the trigeminal ganglion, nerve, or branches
3. Radiofrequency lesioning of the trigeminal ganglion

Both of the trigeminal lesioning techniques (#2 and #3) are reasonably effective but have recurrence problems. Radiofrequency lesioning tends to leave patients with significant facial numbness. Gamma knife procedures are less likely to produce facial sensory loss. The decompression surgery is generally more effective and carries a low risk of both pain recurrence and facial sensation loss. In the hands of experienced surgeons, this procedure has a low mortality rate (<1%) and a high success rate (long-term pain relief up to 80%).

In the case discussed in this chapter, aggressive treatment is indicated. The fact that the patient responded for some time to carbamazepine is a hopeful sign, and a good first step might be to try oxcarbazepine or gabapentin, advancing the dose as tolerated. Nortriptyline might be a good adjunct agent and clonazepam might be another, although all three have the potential to lead to adverse effects. Gabapentin can cause cognitive dysfunction, which is difficult in an elderly patient. Nortriptyline can lead to tachycardia and/or prolonged QT interval, so electrocardiogram monitoring is important. Common adverse effects of dry mouth, constipation, and possibly urine retention can also be frustrating. If prophylactic medication fails, percutaneous gangliolysis might be appropriate here because of its overall safety (no general anesthesia required), but recurrence and facial numbness may be problematic.

KEY POINTS TO REMEMBER

- A number of secondary causes of TN exist, so head MRI is generally indicated.
- Medical treatment of TN is usually successful, with polypharmacy sometimes necessary, limited by adverse effects and medical interactions.
- Surgical options include microvascular decompression and neurolytic procedures.

Further Reading

Bendtsen L, Zakrzewska JM, Abbott J, et al. European Academy of Neurology guideline on trigeminal neuralgia. *Eur J Neurol.* 2019;26:831–849.

Cruccu G. Trigeminal neuralgia. *CONTINUUM.* 2017;23:396–420.

Jannetta PJ. Arterial compression of the trigeminal nerve at the pons in patients with trigeminal neuralgia. *J Neurosurg.* 1967;26:159–162.

Jones MR, Urits I, Ehrhardt KP, et al. A comprehensive review of trigeminal neuralgia. *Curr Pain Headache Rep.* 2019;23:74–81.

18 Acute Treatment of Migraine

Specialties: Neurology, Primary Care, and Communication Skills

It is the first visit for a 27-year-old man, who describes a several-year history of migraine without aura. He reports that his headaches occur three or four times monthly but resolve within 2 hours with 5 mg of oral zolmitriptan. He takes no other medication and has no other significant medical history. As you write his prescription refill, he asks for a medication override, allowing him 18 tablets per month. Perplexed, you inquire why he needs so many pills if he only gets three or four headaches monthly. He tells you that although the medication works quickly, the headache returns either later that day or sometime the next day; this cycle continues for 4 days.

What do you do now?

This case illustrates several important issues. First, it demonstrates the need for clinicians to ask about the number of headache *days* rather than the number of *headaches* per month. To fully ensure that we have truly understood the patient's situation, it can also be very helpful to then go back and ask the opposite question: How many days per month is the patient *completely headache free?* The numbers should add up, and patients should be asked about any days that are unaccounted for. By asking this single question regarding headache-free days, we might end up with a very different picture because many patients, when discussing their symptoms with a clinician, disregard the days in which they have milder head pain, focusing only on their more severe attacks. However, it is important to be fully aware of the complete picture to make an accurate diagnosis. To illustrate, these details can make the difference between understanding that a patient has episodic or chronic migraine, and this can change the entire treatment plan.

Second, this case highlights the need for the clinician to ask about treatment success and to define success in specific terms. A good benchmark for success would be that one dose of the acute medication is well tolerated, terminates the headache pain and associated symptoms of the migraine attack within 2 hours, and that the headache does not return within the next 24 hours.

There are many reasons for treatment refractoriness. Our patient suffers from headache recurrence, the return of an episodic headache during the same migraine attack following the use of an acute treatment. Approximately 20% of triptan users experience a recurrence of their headache 2–24 hours after dosing. For most patients, repeating the same medication will afford relief. In other patients, such as the one described in our case, this cycle can linger for several days with a waxing and waning course. In these instances, the clinician has several options: ensuring that the patient treats the headache early in the attack (within the first 40 minutes of headache onset), that the optimal dose is employed (the highest available dose of the triptan nearly always has a better response), and that the proper formulation is used. For example, oral medications should be avoided in patients with vomiting; nasal spray and parenteral formulations are ideal in this setting. If these measures do not optimize the therapeutic response, additional options include switching to a different triptan (naratriptan and frovatriptan have a lower recurrence rate) or adding a nonsteroidal anti-inflammatory drug

(NSAID), such as naproxen sodium, to the triptan at headache onset. Medication overuse can also occur with triptans: If a patient tells you that a triptan used to be effective in aborting attacks but that the same degree of benefit is no longer experienced, ask about frequency of use. Acute treatment efficacy can certainly be impacted if medication overuse is occurring.

Despite the fact that triptans have revolutionized the acute treatment of migraine, they are not a panacea. As many as 40% of all migraine attacks, and one-fourth of all patients, do not experience benefit from the currently available triptan formulations even after maximizing dose, optimizing route, and ensuring it is taken early in the migraine attack. In these cases, trials of dihydroergotamine, parenterally or intranasally, can sometimes be helpful. In addition, there are data that the new gepants, ubrogepant (Ubrelvy) and rimegepant (Nurtec), can be effective acute treatments in these patients. Consequently, if a person has had an appropriate trial of a few different triptans and has found them ineffective or not tolerated, considering a gepant is an appropriate next choice.

Because triptans are agonists at 5-HT 1B/1D receptors and can potentially cause vasoconstriction, they cannot be used in individuals who have a history of vascular disease or have multiple vascular risk factors. Consequently, there are many people with migraine who are ineligible for triptan therapy. Lasmiditan (Reyvow), a 5-HT 1F agonist approved by the U.S. Food and Drug Administration for the acute treatment of migraine, does not have this potential vascular risk. Gepants are small-molecule antagonists at the calcitonin gene-related peptide receptor that also lack vasoconstrictive activity and can be an option. Navigating between the different gepants and lasmiditan can be tricky, but this can be made simpler by better understanding the patient's personal situation and goals for acute treatment. For example, if a person's ideal scenario is to take their acute treatment, experience quick and complete resolution of the attack, and be able to drive to work, lasmiditan is not a good recommendation because it carries an 8-hour driving restriction due to risks of dizziness. However, if that person's migraine attacks tend to occur in the evening, and their goal is to take their medication and sleep, lasmiditan might be an excellent choice. Rimegepant comes in an oral dissolving formulation, which some patients may prefer or dislike, and ubrogepant should be avoided by those who are on concomitant strong CYP34A inhibitors.

Last, this case may represent a potential candidate for preventive therapy. Just as poor communication between the patient and the clinician can lead to underestimating the disability induced by migraine, so too can it lead to the underutilization of preventive medications. Lipton et al. (2007) reported that approximately 40% of people with migraine are candidates for migraine prevention but only 13% receive treatment. If our patient's headaches continue to be inadequately controlled by the measures discussed previously, he should be prescribed a preventive therapy. In recent years, there has been a shift in the way we consider migraine and when to initiate preventive treatment because it is important not only to consider frequency of attacks, headache days, and acute medication use but also to keep in mind the disability a person experiences from migraine. Even between attacks, migraine can leave an impact, as many people who live with this unpredictable disease understand that the attacks can strike at any moment and plan their day-to-day life accordingly. Furthermore, many people who have migraine are not fully free of symptoms between attacks and have residual photophobia, nausea, mild headache, or other symptoms during this interictal period. Both the disability associated with the attacks and the interictal burden between attacks comprise the total migraine burden. Consequently, even if a person is having infrequent attacks, if their total migraine-related disability is high, starting a preventive medication can be important. Asking questions about the impact migraine has on a person's life and discussing how it has affected their personal, family, social, and work life can not only show our patients we understand their experiences but also help guide treatment decisions.

KEY POINTS TO REMEMBER

- Headache recurrence refers to the return of an episodic headache during the same migraine attack (within 24 hours) following the use of an acute treatment.
- Headache recurrence occurs in approximately 20% of triptan users and usually responds to an additional dose of the same medication.
- Headache recurrence may be lessened by

- treating early in the attack;
- using the highest dose of the triptan;
- avoiding oral formulations in patients who vomit;
- switching to another triptan;
- adding an NSAID to the triptan; and
- switching to dihydroergotamine.
- Gepants and lasmiditan are good options for patients who find triptans ineffective, not tolerated, or have vascular contraindications to triptan therapy.

Further Reading

Ailani J, Burch RC, Robbins MS; Board of Directors of the American Headache Society. The American Headache Society consensus statement: Update on integrating new migraine treatments into clinical practice. *Headache.* 2021;61(7):1021–1039. doi:10.1111/head.14153

Croop R, Goadsby PJ, Stock DA, et al. Efficacy, safety, and tolerability of rimegepant orally disintegrating tablet for the acute treatment of migraine: A randomized, phase 3, double-blind, placebo-controlled trial. *Lancet.* 2019;394(10200):737–745.

Goadsby PJ, Wietecha LA, Dennehy EB, et al. Phase 3 randomized, placebo-controlled, double-blind study of lasmiditan for acute treatment of migraine. *Brain.* 2019;142:1984–1904.

Halker Singh RB, Starling AJ, VanderPluym J. Migraine acute therapies. *Practical Neurol.* 2019 May;65–67.

Kuka B, Silberstein SD, Wietecha L, et al. Lasmiditan is an effective acute treatment for migraine: A phase 3 randomized study. *Neurology.* 2018;91:e2222–e2232.

Lipton RB, Bigal ME, Diamond M, et al. Migraine prevalence, disease burden, and the need for preventive therapy. *Neurology.* 2007;68:343–349.

Lipton RB, Dodick DW, Ailani J, et al. Effect of ubrogepant vs placebo on pain and the most bothersome associated symptom in the acute treatment of migraine: the ACHIEVE II randomized clinical trial. *JAMA.* 2019;322(19):1887–1898.

Marmura MJ, Silberstein SD, Schwedt TJ. The acute treatment of migraine in adults: The American Headache Society evidence assessment of migraine pharmacotherapies. *Headache.* 2015;55(1):3–20.

Pearlman EM, Wilbraham D, Dennehy EB, et al. Effects of lasmiditan on simulated driving performance: Results of two randomized, blinded, crossover studies with placebo and active controls. *Hum Psychopharmacol Clin Exp.* 2020;35:e2732.

Voss T, Lipton RB, Dodick DW, et al. A phase IIb randomized, double-blind, placebo-controlled trial of ubrogepant for the acute treatment of migraine. *Cephalalgia.* 2016;36(9):887–898.

19 Occipital Neuralgia

Approximately 4 months ago, a 32-year-old teacher, while walking down icy steps at school, slipped, fell backward, and struck her occiput. She did not lose consciousness. She experienced moderately severe global headache and neck pain for the next 2 days and then felt well. Approximately 2 or 3 weeks later, she began to experience brief episodes of sharp pain in the right occipital area, which seemed unrelated to movement or position. This pain was not associated with any other symptoms. Pain radiated up the back of the head and to the right vertex. She continues to have this sharp pain and has also developed a significant sensitivity to the right occipital region while brushing her hair, wearing a hat, or laying that side of her head on a pillow. She is otherwise asymptomatic. She does endorse a history of episodic migraine without aura; however, she does insist this pain feels different. Her neurological exam is normal, as is head magnetic resonance imaging (MRI). There is some tenderness in her occiput, and palpation over the right greater occipital notch reproduced her pain and triggered attacks. She is using a large number of ibuprofen and acetaminophen tablets monthly (but she cannot specify the quantity). These analgesics serve only to dull the pain somewhat. Amitriptyline and cyclobenzaprine have not helped. She bursts into tears while relating this history.

What do you do now?

This patient may have post-traumatic headache, but her history and exam suggest occipital neuralgia (ON). This condition can occur after posterior head trauma or whiplash, presumably due to the propensity for damage to the relatively superficial greater occipital nerve (GON), which can easily be compressed against the skull. It has been demonstrated that ON occurs more commonly in patients with other coexisting headache disorders.

The *International Classification of Headache Disorders,* third edition, criteria for diagnosis of ON require that paroxysms of pain occur, variously described as brief (seconds to minutes) or sharp and stabbing strictly localized to one or more of the three occipital nerves—greater, lesser, or third—and either unilateral or bilateral. Furthermore, the criteria requires tenderness, dysesthesia, or allodynia over the emerging symptomatic nerve. Finally, elimination of the pain with a nerve block over the affected nerve is mandatory for diagnosis. Occasionally, the pain may reach to frontal and periorbital locations due to the convergence that occurs at the spinal cord level between nociceptive afferents from anterior head and posterior head regions (trigeminal and upper cervical roots).

Differential diagnosis includes a number of primary and secondary headache disorders: postherpetic neuralgia involving the C2 root or GON; scalp infection or other inflammation; pathological processes involving the upper cervical spine, such as rheumatoid arthritis (or other arthropathy), spinal tumors, or infections of the upper cervical spine; and disorders of the craniocervical junction or posterior cranial fossa, including masses or infections and Chiari I malformation. Occasionally, temporal arteritis involving the occipital artery can mimic some features of ON. Investigation of patients such as this one therefore should usually include inspection of the scalp in the region; cervical spinal examination; imaging of the cervical spine (plain X-ray series might be sufficient); erythrocyte sedimentation rate; and MRI of the head, which should include the craniocervical junction region.

The most useful initial treatment of ON is also diagnostic—anesthetic blockade of the GON. The technique of GON block is relatively simple. The trunk of the GON is located approximately one-third of the distance on a line from the external occipital protuberance to the center of the mastoid. It is adjacent to the occipital artery and can also be located by palpating for this artery. Injection of approximately 1 or 2 cc of 0.25% bupivacaine or 1% lidocaine (or a mixture of the two) in the area of the GON should be sufficient. The GON innervates the scalp from the level of the external occipital protuberance to the vertex on each side, so it is possible to assess the degree of anesthesia by simple sensory testing in the area. The lesser occipital nerve is sometimes involved in the production of pain and can also be blocked with a similar technique and agents.

It seems that clinical benefit is greatest when the area of anesthesia achieved includes the area of the patient's pain. The anesthesia should last for several hours (1 or 2 hours with lidocaine and 4–6 hours with bupivacaine). Surprisingly, this technique can provide relief for patients for much longer—days to weeks or even longer. With this patient's history of heavy use of nonsteroidal anti-inflammatory drugs (NSAIDs), bleeding may complicate the procedure (NSAIDs inhibit platelet aggregation and prolong bleeding time). Other risks of GON blocks include local site infection (rare) and effects of inadvertent intravascular injection such as lightheadedness, tinnitus, anxiety, loss of consciousness, or seizure (unusual because of the low dose of anesthetic and generally easy to avoid by pulling back on the plunger prior to injecting).

If local anesthesia of the GON is effective but pain returns, subsequent GON blocks may prove longer lasting. One can add a corticosteroid such as triamcinolone, although this has not been shown to be any more effective than the local anesthetic agents by themselves. If this is not successful, implantation of a GON stimulator might be warranted. This is costly and carries some minor morbidity risk, but in many cases the benefits are clearly worth the expense and risks. Radiofrequency ablation of the GON may be considered. If pain is refractory, further workup may be appropriate, such as MRI of the cervical spine to search for pathology; C2 root block may also be worth trying. This procedure is slightly more challenging and should be performed under fluoroscopy by trained personnel. However, it can be very effective.

Oral prophylactic medication can help some patients. If the cause of the pain is postherpetic neuralgia, carbamazepine, gabapentin, or pregabalin might be of help. In idiopathic ON, tricyclic antidepressants, anticonvulsants, clonazepam, and NSAIDs have all been helpful in some patients. Muscle relaxants have not proven effective, despite the tender muscle spasm seen in many patients.

Further Reading

Ashkenazi A, Levin M. Nerve blocks and other procedures for headache. In: Silberstein SD, Lipton RB, Dalessio DJ, eds. *Wolff's Headache and Other Head Pain*. 8th ed. New York, NY: Oxford University Press, 2008:Chapter 32, 767–792.

Bogduk N. Role of anesthesiologic blockade in headache management. *Curr Pain Headache Rep*. 2004;8(5):399–403.

Dougherty C. Occipital neuralgia. *Curr Pain Headache Rep*. 2014;18(5):411.

Goadsby PJ, Bartsch T, Dodick DW. Occipital nerve stimulation for headache: Mechanisms and efficacy. *Headache*. 2008;48(2):313–318.

Mathew PG, Najib U, Khaled S, Krel R. Prevalence of occipital neuralgia at a community hospital-based headache clinic. *Neurol. Clin. Pract*. 2021;11:6–12.

20 Headache and Allergy

A 42-year-old woman complains of gradual progression of headaches to daily over the past 5 years. These headaches build in intensity through the morning and generally only resolve when she lies down to go to sleep each evening. They are associated with mild photophobia and nausea. She reports that she has "taken everything out of my diet" (meat, sugar, additives, alcohol, and caffeine) and that this helped somewhat. She believes that she has food and environmental allergies and has tried to avoid as many of these as she can. Skin testing confirmed several of these. She has lactose intolerance and avoids dairy products. She wonders if she has celiac disease. She has seen many physicians, nutritionists, chiropractors, massage therapists, an acupuncturist, and now a craniosacral therapist. No traditional medical therapy "has ever worked," and many medications have led to "horrible" side effects. She refuses to take any pills because of her past experience and because of potential allergens in the colorings in their coatings. The only medication she uses is Excedrin Migraine, which she takes daily, between four and eight tablets.

What do you do now?

This patient likely has chronic migraine, and she seems to be telling you that she is not willing to try any medications whatsoever. However, she does use the acetaminophen–aspirin–caffeine combination, which, by the way, does contain possibly allergenic colorings and excipients. It is also almost certainly leading to medication overuse headache, which can be difficult to prove and even more difficult to reverse if she is unwilling to take any prophylactic medications. This is a tough spot for both the patient and the clinician.

A good first step, as always, is to do what one can to confirm the presumptive diagnosis of primary headache (which type is difficult to determine at this point) with medication overuse overlay. Thorough neurological, head and neck, dental, and general exams should be done. Magnetic resonance imaging of the head will rule out structural lesions, and basic metabolic and hematological screening will rule out such issues as thyroid disease and anemia. Celiac disease, of course, can cause headaches, but usually gastrointestinal symptoms predominate. Serological endomysial antibody screening is a good noninvasive tool, but the gold standard for the diagnosis of celiac disease remains histological confirmation with intestinal biopsy. Another option is to try restriction of wheat and other gluten-containing substances. (Unfortunately, however, it can take several months to see marked improvement.) The food and substance allergies will be equally difficult to confirm because skin testing can be misleading, and a careful plan of dietary restriction may be the only way to proceed (and this is very difficult for patients to accomplish). Perhaps through negotiation with this patient, with help from a nutritionist, you can establish a basic benign diet that can be added to as tolerated while other measures are being pursued.

This patient's fixed ideas about "allopathic" medicine will be an obstacle to helping her improve. What may work best here is to be supportive of the patient's reasonable skepticism of pharmaceutical therapy—it has not worked for her and has led to side effects—but at the same time attempt to convince her that the daily acetaminophen–aspirin–caffeine has to be discontinued. It should be done gradually to avoid caffeine withdrawal. A short course of corticosteroid medication can help patients remain comfortable while attempting to discontinue analgesics. It may be possible to convince this patient to go along with a 10-day course of prednisone beginning with 60 mg for 3 or 4 days and then tapering gradually to zero.

A search for prophylactic and acute medications with little or no coloring may yield some candidates. Several of the cyclic antidepressants and some of the triptans and nonsteroidal anti-inflammatory drugs (NSAIDs) fit these requirements, and with the help of a knowledgeable pharmacist, some acceptable options may emerge. Neuromodulation devices may be of particular benefit in these cases.

As for additional nonpharmacological treatment, there is a plethora to choose from and this is the problem. No patient has the time to systematically try all of the "complementary and alternative" options for headaches. Fortunately, there is evidence for the usefulness of several modalities, including relaxation techniques, cognitive–behavioral therapy, and thermal and electromyographic biofeedback (Box 20.1). Acupuncture, hypnotherapy, and massage therapy have some scientific support. Of the vitamin and herbal therapies, magnesium, coenzyme Q$_{10}$, riboflavin (vitamin B$_2$), and feverfew (leaf) are supported by some evidence. Chiropractic treatment has yet to be shown to be effective for headaches. The so-called energy therapies, including reiki, craniosacral therapy, qi gong, and meditation, are also proposed widely, but scientific support is not yet available.

KEY POINTS TO REMEMBER

- Over-the-counter medications such as NSAIDs and, in particular, combination medications such as acetaminophen–aspirin–caffeine can lead to medication overuse headache, which can mimic chronic migraine.

- Food and other environmental allergies are rarely causes of headaches in the absence of other symptoms.
- Nonpharmacological therapies that are evidence-based include cognitive–behavioral therapy, relaxation techniques, and biofeedback. Biofeedback and massage have some scientific support.
- Herbal/vitamin headache therapies that have some scientific support include magnesium, vitamin B_2, feverfew, butterbur, and coenzyme Q_{10}.

Further Reading

Holroyd KA, Mauskop A. Complementary and alternative treatments. *Neurology.* 2003;60(Suppl.):s58–s62.

Levin, M. Herbal treatment of headache. *Headache.* 2012;52(Suppl. 2):76–80.

Martin V, Vij B. Diet and headache: Part 1. Headache. *J Head Face Pain.* 2016;56(9):1543–1552.

Razeghi Jahromi S, Ghorbani Z, Martelletti P, Lampl C, Togha M; School of Advanced Studies of the European Headache Federation. Association of diet and headache. *J Headache Pain.* 2019;20:106.

Vickers AJ, Rees RW, Zollman CE, et al. Acupuncture for chronic headache in primary care: Large, pragmatic, randomised trial. *BMJ.* 2004;328:744–750.

21 Headache Treatment in Human Immunodeficiency Virus Infection

A 62-year-old man with human immunodeficiency virus (HIV) but normal white blood cell counts on antiretroviral agents has four or five severe headaches per week that respond only minimally to over-the-counter acetaminophen. These headaches have been present "for years," are generally unilateral and throbbing, and can be accompanied by nausea and photophobia. Several prophylactic medications have not worked, including amitriptyline, duloxetine, topiramate, and propranolol. He also carries a diagnosis of coronary artery disease s/p coronary artery bypass grafting and has aortic valve stenosis s/p St. Jude's valve insertion and is on warfarin. He also has chronically elevated liver enzyme levels secondary to fatty liver disease and suffers from chronic constipation. Magnetic resonance imaging (MRI) without and with gadolinium performed 2 months ago was negative. Exam is unremarkable.

What do you do now?

This case would challenge a seasoned headache specialist. What often works best in complex headache cases is to break them down into components. Here, the key questions revolve around (1) diagnosis, (2) choices for acute relief of migraine when triptans are contraindicated, and (3) preventive medication options when numerous options have failed and comorbidities exist.

Regarding diagnosis, although migraine is most likely, there are a number of other possibilities that should be considered. In this case, the MRI reassuringly speaks against intracranial infection or neoplasm. He presumably has no signs of meningeal irritation, so meningitis as a cause of headaches is unlikely as well. However, given his history of being immunocompromised with HIV, if there are any remaining concerns of an infectious or inflammatory process, lumbar puncture should be pursued. The virus can cause headaches itself, perhaps on the basis of active central nervous system (CNS) infection or due to the fact that the metabolism of serotonin and tryptophan seems to be altered in HIV infection. Antivirals used in HIV-infected patients can lead to headaches as well. However, Mirsattari et al. (1999) found that primary headaches in patients with HIV infection are very common and usually not related to the antiretroviral drug therapy. They concluded that many cases do not require neuroradiological and/or cerebrospinal fluid examination.

If workup is unrevealing and exam remains stable, it is appropriate to treat this man's headaches as chronic migraine. Preventive treatment is indicated due to the frequency and the recurring need for analgesia. Although he is on anticoagulation, Botox treatment may be the most reasonable next therapeutic option to offer. To date, there has been no reported increased risk of bleeding complications for patients on antithrombotic therapy who receive Botox treatment. Nonetheless, patient education and careful observation of the injection site should be undertaken. Calcitonin gene-related peptide (CGRP) monoclonal antibodies may also be considered; however, given the potential for these to contribute to constipation in a patient in whom this is already a comorbidity, caution is advisable.

In general, beta-blockers, tricyclic antidepressants, topiramate, and perhaps calcium channel blockers can make good choices in patients with HIV naïve to headache prophylactic treatment; but there are risks. Beta-blockers should be used with caution with atazanavir because of the tendency for both to prolong the P–R interval. Ritonavir and other protease inhibitors suppress some hepatic enzyme systems [e.g., cytochrome P-450 3A4 (CYP 3A4)], which could elevate other medication levels (e.g., calcium channel blockers as well as ergots and eletriptan). There is some evidence that valproate may lead to increased replication of HIV. Finally, topiramate induces CYP 3A4 and, thus, can decrease protease inhibitor levels with possible reactivation of the HIV infection.

As for nontriptan acute antimigraine agents, anti-nausea medications such as promethazine (Phenergan) 25 mg po or suppository or metoclopramide (Reglan) 10 mg po might prove effective here. NSAIDs should be used with caution given coronary artery disease history. This patient would be an excellent candidate for some of the newer migraine treatment options, including lasmitidan in addition to CGRP receptor antagonists such as ubrogepant and rimegepant. Neuromodulation devices are a very appropriate option for acute treatment as well and could include Cefaly® and Nerivio Migra®.

KEY POINTS TO REMEMBER

- There are several ways that HIV can lead to headaches: (1) a direct consequence of the CNS HIV infection (perhaps due to neurotransmitter alteration); (2) opportunistic infections of the head and neck, including meningitis and cerebral toxoplasmosis; (3) intracranial neoplasms; and (4) as an adverse effect of antiretroviral or other medications used to treat HIV or HIV-related disease.
- One should carefully consider medication interactions as well as comorbidities when choosing the most appropriate acute and preventive medications in HIV patients on antiretroviral medications.

Further Reading

Dimitrova R, James L, Liu C, Orejudos A, Yushmanova I, Brin MF. Safety of onabotulinumtoxinA with concomitant antithrombotic therapy in patients with muscle spasticity: A retrospective pooled analysis of randomized double-blind studies. *CNS Drugs*. 2020;34:433–445.

Dodick D, Lipton RB, Martin V, et al. Consensus statement: Cardiovascular safety profile of triptans (5-HT1B/1D agonists) in the acute treatment of migraine. *Headache*. 2004;44:414–425.

Goldstein J. Headache and acquired immunodeficiency syndrome. *Neurol Clin*. 1990;8:947–960.

Joshi SG, Cho TA. Pathophysiological mechanisms of headache in patients with HIV. *Headache*. 2014;54(5):946–950.

Kirkland KE, Kirkland K, Many WJ Jr, Smitherman TA. Headache among patients with HIV disease: Prevalence, characteristics and associations. *Headache*. 2011;52(3):455–466.

Mirsattari S, Power C, Nath A. Primary headaches in HIV-infected patients. *Headache*. 1999;39:3–10.

22 Idiopathic Intracranial Hypertension

A 32-year-old obese woman began having global aching and throbbing headaches last year that were unassociated with nausea, vomiting, or photophobia. She reports occasional pulsatile tinnitus. Papilledema was noted after several months but has lessened more recently. Magnetic resonance imaging (MRI) of the brain was normal, as were neurological and general exams. Lumbar puncture (LP) revealed an opening pressure of 28 cm of H_2O. Cerebrospinal fluid (CSF) was acellular and otherwise normal. She did not notice an improvement in head pain after LP. A second LP revealed an opening pressure of 31 cm of H_2O. She is using ibuprofen, acetaminophen, and hydrocodone nearly daily. Acetazolamide has caused unpleasant paresthesias in her hands and feet at the current dose of 500 mg daily, and she has had little improvement in headache.

What do you do now?

Pseudotumor cerebri, literally meaning "false tumor," is a condition in which the pressure inside the skull is increased. Many secondary causes have been associated with pseudotumor cerebri, such as medications, endocrine disorders, and obstructive sleep apnea. When no secondary cause is identified, the syndrome is termed "idiopathic intracranial hypertension" (IIH). IIH is seen predominantly in obese women of childbearing age. Proposed pathophysiological mechanisms include CSF hypersecretion, CSF outflow obstruction (dysfunction in arachnoid granulations), or increase in venous sinus pressure. The presentation is usually fairly pathognomonic—headache, papilledema, and pulsatile tinnitus. Papilledema can be asymmetrical, and some patients do not develop it. Occasionally, some radicular pain in the upper extremities is reported, and some patients experience transient visual obscurations. The LP opening pressure should be above 25 cm. Sixth nerve palsies can occur with symptoms of horizontal diplopia. Visual field testing can reveal an enlarged blind spot. An MRI scan of the head is generally normal, although empty sella, flattening of the globes posteriorly, tortuosity of the optic nerves, and small ("slit-like") ventricles can be seen. Several medications have been implicated in the genesis of intracranial hypertension, including vitamin A–related compounds (e.g., isotretinoin and Accutane), corticosteroids, cimetidine, thyroid medications, estrogenic medications, lithium, and tetracycline.

After MRI rules out mass lesions and hydrocephalus, as it did in this patient, other possibilities include lupus, lupus anticoagulant syndrome, Lyme disease (as well as other chronic meningitides such as tuberculosis, syphilis, and *Cryptococcus* infection), cerebral venous thrombosis, and leukemia. Magnetic resonance venography is indicated in all patients with atypical presentations (men, children, and those with low body mass index) because a number of patients diagnosed with IIH have later been shown to have occlusion of one or more cerebral veins. Thyroid and other hormonal abnormalities have been implicated as well, so thyroid-stimulating hormone, growth hormone, anti-nuclear antibodies, lupus anticoagulant, anti-cardiolipin antibody, VDRL, Lyme titer, complete blood count, and perhaps HIV testing should be done. Pregnancy is said to be a risk factor for the development of IIH; therefore, a pregnancy test is worthwhile in all potentially pregnant patients.

In cases such as this one, the first step is to ensure the workup is negative. Next, you need to convince yourself this is really IIH, rather than a primary chronic daily headache. For example, was the LP done in the lateral decubitus position? (If done sitting or even prone, as is typical in fluoroscopically guided LPs, the opening pressure can be falsely elevated. If anesthesia was used or the patient had any Valsalva activities, such as crying during procedure, the opening pressure can also be falsely elevated.) Migraine features are not present here, but they may have been missed. Medication overuse headache can complicate the picture as well. The papilledema and high opening pressures (if accurate) would seem compelling for the diagnosis of IIH in our case, at least for now.

Thus, there are really only two concerns at this point: (1) pain control and (2) prevention of visual compromise, the only actual morbidity encountered in IIH. Monitoring of visual acuity and visual fields by an ophthalmological consultant is therefore essential. Ocular ultrasound as well as optical coherence testing can further help diagnose papilledema versus drusen or congenital disc anomalies. These techniques are also very helpful for monitoring impact of treatment over time. If there has been evidence of rapid or progressive visual loss, more urgent management should be taken. Prednisone can reduce CSF pressure and papilledema, in doses of 60–80 mg daily for exacerbations. Long-term treatment is risky, so corticosteroids are usually reserved for exacerbations. If deterioration in vision occurs, optic nerve sheath fenestration (ONF) should be considered. This usually preserves vision, but recurrence of visual impairment can happen later, so this must be followed. Headaches do not generally improve with ONF.

Headache often does not respond to acetazolamide, as seen in this patient, and many patients find it intolerable. The addition of furosemide may help reduce headaches and might be an option here, which might allow a decrease in acetazolamide. As long as visual acuity is stable, experimenting with medications used for treating primary headaches is reasonable. For example, amitriptyline or nortriptyline, topiramate (which has some carbonic anhydrase inhibiting activity itself, like acetazolamide), other anticonvulsants, and beta-blockers are worth considering. Headaches do not seem to improve after LP, but lumboperitoneal shunting is still sometimes used despite the fact that complications are frequent (e.g., dislodgment or other failure of shunt and infection). Venous sinus stenting has also been used recently with varying results.

Finally, because obesity is clearly a risk factor for IIH, weight loss in obese patients such as this one is considered a key treatment goal. When patients are unable to accomplish this, gastric bypass is a real consideration, when either headaches or visual effects are intractable.

KEY POINTS TO REMEMBER

- Idiopathic intracranial hypertension is most likely to occur in young obese women but can occur in other groups as well.
- Diagnosing IIH is based on elevated CSF pressure as well as the characteristic features of global headache, pulsatile tinnitus, and papilledema.
- Differential diagnosis includes cerebral venous thrombosis, so MRI should also include venography in atypical cases.
- Lupus and endocrinological disease can lead to increased intracranial pressure, so rheumatological and hormonal workup is also worthwhile.
- The only morbidity in IIH is preventable visual loss, so close monitoring of visual acuity and visual fields is imperative.

Further Reading

Farb RI, Vanek I, Scott JN, et al. Idiopathic intracranial hypertension: The prevalence and morphology of sinovenous stenosis. *Neurology.* 2003;60(9):1418–1424.

Friedman DI. Idiopathic intracranial hypertension. *Curr Pain Headache Rep.* 2007;11:62–68.

Markey KA, Mollan SP, Jensen RH, Sinclair AJ. Understanding idiopathic intracranial hypertension: Mechanisms, management, and future directions. *Lancet Neurol.* 2016;15:78–91.

Smith S, Friedman D. The Idiopathic Intracranial Hypertension Treatment Trial: A review of the outcomes. *Headache.* 2017;57(8):1303–1310.

23 Postdural Puncture Headache

A 72-year-old man was referred to you by his orthopedist. He complains of a 2-week history of daily, unremitting headaches beginning 3 days after a knee replacement. The surgery was performed with spinal anesthesia and a regional nerve block. The headaches are described as sharp, pressure-like with occasional throbbing, are of moderate to severe intensity, and are located at the vertex, temples, and retro-orbitally. He reports that when severe, the headaches are associated with photo- and phonophobia, fatigue, and lightheadedness. He denies any positional component and states that he has been awakened from sleep by the head pain on several nights. Oral nonsteroidal anti-inflammatory drugs have not relieved the pain, but intravenous ketorolac given in the emergency department reduced the pain to a significant degree but only for a few hours. Magnetic resonance imaging (MRI) of the brain with and without contrast, a sedimentation rate, C-reactive protein, and Lyme titer obtained during his emergency department visit were normal. He has no prior history of headaches.

What do you do now?

Headaches following spinal anesthesia should raise concern for a postdural puncture headache (PDPH). PDPH may be the result of a lumbar puncture, myelogram, or an inadvertent dural puncture during neuraxial anesthesia. Risk factors for developing PDPH include younger age, female gender, prior headache history, low body mass index, large bore or cutting needle, and the use of air rather than saline as a means of measuring resistance during epidural catheter placement.

The incidence of headache following dural puncture has been reported in the obstetric literature (D'Angelo et al. 2014). Postdural headaches occurred in 1 out of 144 neuraxial anesthetic procedures (spinal anesthesia and accidental dural punctures during epidural anesthesia), so it was not possible to determine the number of true accidental dural punctures. However, of the 1,674 patients who reported headaches, 56% required one blood patch and 11% required two patches.

The characteristic clinical feature of PDPH is headache often positional in nature, worsening within 15 minutes of assuming an upright position, and improving when the patient reclines. The longer the patient has remained upright, the longer it takes for the headache to resolve with recumbency. Although orthostatic headaches are classic for this syndrome, other non-orthostatic presentations, as described by our patient, are possible. These headaches are usually throbbing, bilateral, localized to the occipital or suboccipital areas, and worsened with Valsalva maneuvers. The headaches may be associated with nausea, dizziness, neck pain or stiffness, tinnitus, hypacusia, photophobia, intrascapular pain, nausea, vomiting, blurred vision, and diplopia (secondary to cranial nerve palsies) (Graff-Radford and Schievink 2014). The *International Classification of Headache Disorders,* third edition, criteria for headaches attributed to low cerebrospinal fluid (CSF) pressure and headaches following dural puncture are listed in Boxes 23.1 and 23.2.

PDPH results from decreased CSF volume from a leak at the dural puncture site, which causes sinking of the brain in the skull. This "brain sag" induces traction on the pain-sensitive suspending and anchoring structures of the brain and is responsible for the headaches and associated signs and symptoms of this disorder. The positional component of the headache (when present) is the result of the increase in the downward displacement of the brain and the increase in traction upon the pain-sensitive structures

that occurs in a gravity-dependent manner when the patient assumes an
upright position. Traction upon cranial nerves III–VIII and the brainstem
results in nerve palsies and mental status changes, whereas the changes in
pressure that are transmitted into the perilymphatic fluid produce the tinnitus, hypacusia, and vestibular symptoms.

In most cases, the diagnosis of PDPH is established by history. Patients report the typical orthostatic headache beginning within 5 days of a procedure
that deliberately or inadvertently punctures the dura. Lumbar puncture to
document low opening pressures is generally not advised in these situations
because it can worsen the symptomatology. In cases in which there are atypical features, or the disorder is chronic and unrelenting, further evaluation is
warranted. Brain MRI without gadolinium may demonstrate brain sag, descent of the cerebellar tonsils (pseudo-Chiari I), a decrease in the prepontine

or perichiasmatic cisterns, flattening of the optic chiasm, posterior fossa crowding, a decrease in the size of the ventricles, subdural collections, and enlargement of the venous sinuses. MRI with contrast is the procedure of choice in these circumstances and typically shows diffuse pachymeningeal, but not leptomeningeal, enhancement. This finding is not always present and may disappear over time; therefore, it is not required for the diagnosis.

Because symptoms can spontaneously remit in the majority of patients within 2 weeks, the treatment of PDPH includes conservative measures such as bed rest and hydration, simple analgesics, and caffeine administration (by mouth or intravenously). If conservative measures fail, or in cases in which the pain and disability are high, epidural blood patching, in which the patient is injected with 10–30 mL of autologous blood into the epidural space at the site of the prior procedure, should be performed. Some patients require more than one patch for relief. When repeated blood patches fail, percutaneous placement of 4–20 mL of fibrin sealant injected via a foraminal approach may offer relief. For refractory cases, surgical exploration and dural repair are necessary.

Our patient had new-onset headache following a surgical procedure in which spinal anesthesia was used. Although his headaches were not orthostatic and his contrast-enhanced MRI was normal, neither are diagnostic criteria, and they should not eliminate PDPH as the diagnosis. The emergency department physicians were correct to search for other culprits of new-onset headache in the elderly. Because all prior testing was normal and the patient was in extreme pain, a blood patch was performed, which resulted in immediate and sustained headache relief.

KEY POINTS TO REMEMBER

- Postdural puncture headache occurs within 5 days of a procedure that deliberately or accidently penetrates the dura.
- Headache is typically, but not always, orthostatic.
- Neuroimaging may be normal or may show "brain sag" or pachymeningeal enhancement.
- Risk factors include female gender, younger age, low body mass index, prior headache history, and the use of large-bore or cutting needles.
- If conservative treatments fail, blood patching is warranted.

Further Reading

D'Angelo R, Smiley RM, Riley ET, et al. Serious complications related to obstetric anesthesia: The Serious Complication Repository Project of the Society for Obstetric Anesthesia and Perinatology. *Anesthesiology.* 2014;120:1505–1512.

Gaiser RR. Postdural puncture headache: An evidence-based approach. *Anesthesiology Clin.* 2017;35:157–167.

Graff-Radford SB, Schievink WI. High-pressure headaches, low-pressure headaches, and CSF leaks: Diagnosis and treatment. *Headache.* 2014;54:394–401.

International Classification Committee of the International Headache Society. The *International Classification of Headache Disorders*, 3rd edition. *Cephalalgia.* 2018;38:1–211.

Smith JH, Mac Grory B, Butterfield RJ, et al. CSF pressure, volume, and post-dural puncture headache: A case–control study and systematic review. *Headache.* 2019;59:1324–1338.

24 Refractory Chronic Migraine

A 46-year-old woman with a 10-year history of unremitting headaches presents to your office for the first time. She describes, and a review of her medical records confirms, a history of migraine that began at age 15 years and has steadily increased in frequency during the past two decades. She has been treated with several antidepressants, anticonvulsants, and antihypertensive classes at the appropriate doses and duration, and in multiple combinations, without significant improvement. For the past year, she has been receiving onabotulinumtoxinA (Botox) injections every 12 weeks, which has decreased her headache frequency from 30 to 15 days monthly. A review of her headache diary reveals that severe, unrelenting migraines occur 2 weeks before her next round of her medication is due, during which time she requires treatment in the emergency department on at least 4 of those days.

What do you do now?

Chronic migraine (CM) is defined as >15 headache days/month for more than 3 months, and on at least 8 days/month the headache has the features of migraine headache (Box 24.1). It is estimated that CM affects 1.4–2.2% of the global population. Bigal and colleagues have reported that approximately 2.5% of people with episodic migraine (EM) transform into the chronic form every year. Not surprisingly, CM has been shown to cause greater headache-related disability, headache impact, societal burden, and lower quality of life scores compared with EM.

In general, all patients with CM require preventive therapy. The goals of and indications for preventive treatments are listed in Boxes 24.2 and 24.3. Most of the preventive medications employed in the treatment of migraine are off-label. Only six medications (topiramate, divalproex sodium, propranolol, atogepant, and rimegepant timolol) are approved by the U.S. Food and Drug Administration for the treatment of EM, and only onabotulinumtoxin A (OBTA) is approved for the prevention of CM. The four injectable monoclonal antibodies (mAbs) that target calcitonin gene-related peptide (CGRP)—erenumab, fremanezumab, galcanezumab, and eptinezumab—are approved for migraine prevention; their use is not limited based on headache frequency.

In clinical trials, a >50% reduction in the mean number of monthly headache days (MHD) is the standard by which most medications are

---

BOX 24.1 **ICHD-3 Criteria for Chronic Migraine**

A. Migraine-like or tension-type-like headache on ≥15 days/month for >3 months that fulfills criteria B and C
B. Occurring in a patient who has had at least five attacks fulfilling criteria B–D for migraine without aura and/or criteria B and C for migraine with aura
C. On ≥8 days/month for >3 months, fulfilling any of the following:
   1. Criteria C and D for migraine without aura
   2. Criteria B and C for migraine with aura
   3. Believed by the patient to be migraine at onset and relieved by a triptan or ergot derivative
D. Not better accounted for by another diagnosis

ICHD-3, *International Classification of Headache Disorders*, third edition.

deemed efficacious. Although this may be a useful parameter for gauging success in a trial, in real life this is not an optimal outcome for many patients with CM. Consider the patient with 15 MHD: Reducing their attack days by half allows them to live most of the month headache-free, yet for those with daily headaches, such as the patient discussed in this chapter, that same 50% reduction means they continue to live with CM.

Many patients receiving treatment with OBTA experience a "wearing off" of the beneficial effects before their next dose is due, often within the last 2 weeks. Kahn et al. (2019) found that 44% of their patients reported worsening of their headaches or neck pain in the 28 days prior to their next dose. Masters-Israilov and Robbins (2019) reported that wear-off occurred in 63% of patients treated with OBTA for CM, with breakthrough pain most often occurring 2–4 weeks before the next injections were scheduled. Because OBTA injections are given at 12-week intervals, this suggests that for a sizable proportion of patients, the beneficial effects only last approximately two-thirds of the dosing period. Zidan et al. (2019) studied the variation in weekly headache frequency during the 12-week period following treatment with OBTA for CM. They found that the time–response plot had three distinct phases, each lasting 4 weeks: an induction phase, in which headache frequency declined rapidly; a maximum efficacy phase between weeks 4 and 8 during which the headache frequency stabilized; and a wearing-off phase beginning at week 8 post-injection, during which time the headache frequency increased to the baseline frequency.

There are several options to combat the end-of-dosing loss of efficacy. The simplest option is to increase the dose of OBTA administered at each 12-week session. Although the standard dose employed is 155 units given in 31 fixed sites as suggested from the PREEMPT studies, these studies permitted the physician to use an additional 40 units at their discretion [up to eight additional injections (each of 5 units) could be administered in up to three specific muscle areas (occipitalis, temporalis, and trapezius)]. There have not been any head-to-head trials comparing these two doses, yet in the office setting, many clinicians have noted that higher doses may increase the duration of the therapeutic effect of OBTA, using the "follow-the-pain" paradigm.

Another strategy is to perform occipital (see Chapter 19) or sphenopalatine nerve blocks at the 10-week mark, when OBTA efficacy begins to wane. Adding an oral migraine preventive agent to OBTA may potentially prevent or lessen the impact of the wearing-off effect. Combining one of the injectable CGRP mAbs to OBTA therapy would be a rational therapeutic approach because most patients would not have previously tried these agents before initiating OBTA treatment, whereas they would have been required by most insurers to have tried and failed several of the standard oral migraine preventives before being approved for OBTA treatment. Unfortunately, in our experience, most payers do not permit this combination, based ostensibly on the lack of studies using the combination but more realistically based on the cost.

Alternatively, administering the OBTA dose every 10 weeks would mitigate the wearing-off phenomenon; however, in our experience, most insurers balk at this increased dosing frequency and refuse to cover the cost of the additional yearly treatment.

Our patient was treated by increasing her dose of ONTA to 195 units every 12 weeks, which successfully eliminated her breakthrough headaches and reduced her headache frequency to 6 days monthly. Should her headache frequency increase again in the future, then one of the other options will be explored.

KEY POINTS TO REMEMBER

· A large proportion of patients treated with OBTA experience wearing off of the beneficial effects 2–4 weeks prior to the next scheduled injection cycle.
· Bridge therapies include occipital nerve or sphenopalatine nerve blocks at the 10-week mark.
· Increasing the OBTA dose from 155 units to 195 units or redosing at 10 rather than 12 weeks may prevent wear-off.
· Adding oral preventive medications or injectable CGRP mAbs to the OBTA may reduce migraine attacks.

Further Reading

Ailani J, Burch RC, Robbins MS; Board of Directors of the American Headache Society. The American Headache Society consensus statement: Update on integrating new migraine treatments into clinical practice. *Headache*. 2021;61:1021–1039.

Bigal ME, Serrano D, Reed M, Lipton RB. Chronic migraine in the population: Burden, diagnosis, and satisfaction with treatment. *Neurology*. 2008;71:559–566.

Dodick DW, Turkel CC, DeGryse RE, et al. OnabotulinumtoxinA for treatment of chronic migraine: Pooled results from the double-blind, randomized, placebo-controlled phases of the PREEMPT clinical program. *Headache*. 2010;50:921–936.

Kahn FA, Mohammed AE, Poogkunran M, et al. Wearing off effect of onabotulinumtoxinA near the end of treatment cycle for chronic migraine: A 4-year clinical experience. *Headache*. 2019;60:430–440.

Masters-Israilov A, Robbins MS. OnabotulinumtoxinA wear-off phenomenon in the treatment of chronic migraine. *Headache*. 2019;59:1753–1761.

Zidan A, Roe C, Burke D, Mejico L. OnabotulinumtoxinA wear-off in chronic migraine, observational cohort study. *J Clin Neurosci*. 2019;69:237–240.

25 High-Altitude Headache

Specialties: Neurology, Sports and Exercise Medicine, and Primary Care

A 37-year-old man presents for an office visit. He states that he went hiking in the Rocky Mountains on a recent family trip and developed a moderately severe bilateral throbbing headache during the ascent. With the headache, he also experienced nausea, dizziness, fatigue, and shortness of breath. It only improved after returned back home to Florida. He has another similar trip planned with a group of friends, and he wants to know what he can do to keep this from happening again. He does not regularly get headaches.

What do you do now?

The *International Classification of Headache Disorders*, third edition (ICHD-3), categorizes high-altitude headache (HAH) as a disorder of homeostasis. It tends to occur when ascending altitudes higher than 2500 m and resolves within 24 hours of descending to less than 2500 m. More than 30% of mountaineers will experience a headache at elevations, particularly with rapid ascent and at very high altitudes. HAH can accompany acute mountain sickness (AMS), with other symptoms part of this syndrome being nausea, fatigue, dizziness, loss of appetite, dyspnea, and sleep disturbance. Having a personal history of migraine, a high perceived degree of physical exertion, dehydration (<2 L in 24 hours), restrictions in venous outflow, and low arterial oxygen saturation are all risk factors for HAH. Because migraine is associated with HAH, there can be quite a bit of clinical overlap between the two. However, with HAH, the presence of a unilateral pain location, photophobia, and phonophobia would be atypical (Box 25.1).

From a pathophysiology standpoint, cellular hypoxia as a result of decreased barometric pressure at higher elevations appears to be a critical factor. The brain is exquisitely sensitive to hypoxia, and if AMS is allowed

---

BOX 25.1 **ICHD-3 Diagnostic Criteria for High-Altitude Headache**

A. Headache fulfilling criterion C
B. Ascent to altitude above 2500 m has occurred.
C. Evidence of causation demonstrated by at least two of the following:
  1. Headache has developed in temporal relation to the ascent.
  2. Either or both of the following:
    a. Headache has significantly worsened in parallel with continuing ascent.
    b. Headache has resolved within 24 hours after descent to below 2500 m.
  3. Headache has at least two of the following three characteristics:
    a. Bilateral location
    b. Mild or moderate intensity
    c. Aggravated by exertion, movement, straining coughing, and/ or bending
D. Not better accounted for by another ICHD-3 diagnosis

ICHD-3, *International Classification of Headache Disorders*, third edition.

---

to progress, individuals can develop symptoms of high-altitude cerebral edema, such as confusion, gait ataxia, personality changes, and alterations in levels of consciousness.

From a preventive standpoint, allowing at least 24-48 hours for acclimatization during ascents can be helpful in preventing HAH, as can liberalizing fluid intake and avoiding alcohol. Obviously, as per diagnostic criteria, descent from high altitude should lead to spontaneous headache resolution within 24 hours. Because cellular hypoxia is a causative factor for HAH, oxygen supplementation can also be helpful, and the headache should resolve after 10–15 minutes of supplemental oxygen therapy. For milder HAH, simple analgesics, such as acetaminophen and ibuprofen, can also give pain relief. Medications that suppress respiratory drive should be avoided, including opiates, benzodiazepines, barbiturates, and others that can be sedating.

There is evidence that acetazolamide (125–250 mg twice daily) is effective for AMS prevention and acute therapy, and it can be started the day prior to ascent. Acetazolamide is a carbonic anhydrase inhibitor that can lead to metabolic acidosis. Its role in the treatment of AMS may be related to the fact that it also decreases cerebrospinal fluid production.

Dexamethasone, a corticosteroid that reduces capillary permeability by inhibiting cytokine release, can be used acutely to treat high-altitude cerebral edema. Nifedipine, a calcium channel blocker, as well as phosphodiesterase 5 inhibitors, such as sildenafil and tadalafil, can treat pulmonary hypertension and therefore decrease high-altitude-induced pulmonary edema.

Relatedly, airplane headache (AH) is a new diagnosis introduced in ICHD-3 (Box 25.2). This head pain is described as a severe, unilateral, periorbital headache, with a stabbing, jabbing, or pulsating quality, associated with airplane travel. More than 90% of cases occur during airplane descent rather than during takeoff. It generally resolves within 30 minutes of landing. Although the pathophysiology behind this headache is unclear, sinus barotrauma as well as a discrepancy between intrasinus and external air pressures have been implicated as potential causative factors. Individuals with AH can experience associated symptoms, most often restlessness and unilateral tearing. Chewing, extending the earlobe, and applying pressure to the painful area can sometimes be helpful. There have also been reports of naproxen, ibuprofen, and triptans being used for AH.

ICHD-3 Criteria for Headache Attributed to Airplane Travel

A. At least two episodes of headache fulfilling criterion C
B. The patient is traveling by airplane.
C. Evidence of causation demonstrated by at least two of the following:
  1. Headache has developed during the airplane flight.
  2. Either or both of the following:
    a. Headache has worsened in temporal relation to ascent following takeoff and/or descent prior to landing of the airplane.
    b. Headache has spontaneously improved within 30 minutes after the ascent or descent of the airplane is completed.
  3. Headache is severe, with at least two of the following three characteristics:
    a. Unilateral location
    b. Orbitofrontal location
    c. Jabbing or stabbing quality
D. Not better accounted for by another ICHD-3 diagnosis

ICHD-3, *International Classification of Headache Disorders*, third edition.

KEY POINTS TO REMEMBER

- High-altitude headache is common, and it can occur in more than 30% of mountaineers.
- A personal history of migraine, a high perceived degree of physical exertion, dehydration (<2 L in 24 hours), restrictions in venous outflow, and low arterial oxygen saturation are all risk factors for HAH.
- From a preventive standpoint, allowing at least 24–48 hours for acclimatization during ascents can be helpful in preventing HAH, as can allowing for liberal fluid intake and avoiding alcohol.
- Acetazolamide (125–250 mg twice daily) is effective for AMS prevention and acute therapy, and it can be started the day prior to ascent.

Further Reading

Joshi SG, Mechtler LL. Sherpas, coca leaves, and planes: High altitude and airplane headache review with a case of post-LASIK myopic shift. *Curr Neurol Neurosci Rep.* 2019;19(12):104. doi:10.1007/s11910-019-1013-0

Lopez JI, Holdridge A, Mendizabal JE. Altitude headache. *Curr Pain Headache Rep.* 2013;17(12):383.

Luks AM, Swenson ER, Bärtsch P. Acute high-altitude sickness. *Eur Respir Rev.* 2017;26(143):160096.

Marmura MJ, Hernandez PB. High-altitude headache. *Curr Pain Headache Rep.* 2015;19(5):483.

Headache Treatment
in Depression and Anxiety

A 20-year-old college student is referred for an increasing migraine frequency that has become disabling to the point of negatively impacting her academic performance. She endorses near daily pain that is unilateral and throbbing, associated with nausea, lethargy, and significant photophobia. In the past year, she has also developed visual symptoms preceding her migraine described as a shiny "C-shaped" ring that lasts approximately 20 minutes with a subsequent typical migraine following. The first time this occurred, she was so frightened that she went to the local emergency department, where she had an ophthalmology exam and magnetic resonance imaging of her brain, both of which were unremarkable. Her neurological exam is normal. However, her affect is depressed, and she becomes tearful when describing the impact her migraines have had on her life. She states that they are so bad that sometimes she "just doesn't want to wake up." She has also gained 15 pounds in the past year, which she thinks may be due to inability to exercise due to headaches. She endorses a history of feeling sad when she was younger; however, she has difficulty recalling the details and she states she had a "very difficult childhood" and her father was an alcoholic. She has never seen a psychiatrist or been formally diagnosed with a mood disorder.

What do you do now?

Psychiatric comorbidities are commonly seen in headache patients and can pose both opportunities and challenges for treatment. It has been postulated that headaches are not just a symptom of depression or anxiety, but that headaches and mood disorders share a number of pathophysiological similarities, including dysfunction of neurotransmitters and hypothalamic–pituitary–adrenal axis dysregulation. It is crucial to screen for psychiatric comorbidities in all headache patients because these seems to increase the risk of development of headache chronicity, decrease quality of life, and complicate management. Of utmost importance is to recognize a patient who may be at risk for harm to themself or others, which is a significant concern in the patient described.

The most common mood disorders seen in headache patients include depression, anxiety and bipolar disorder. Personality disorders have been less well characterized in the headache literature, but when present, they are clearly complicating factors in headache management. Abuse and post-traumatic stress disorder (PTSD) are also frequently seen in migraine patients (as opposed to tension headache) and should be addressed. This patient described a "difficult childhood" suggestive of abuse. Treating PTSD alone could improve the sense of well-being and significantly reduce pain and disability in patients with migraine. Migraine has also been associated with substance abuse, nicotine dependence, and illicit drug use (see Chapter 27). Sleep disorders such as insomnia are also commonly seen.

Screening for comorbid psychiatric disease is recommended in all headache patients. Although some clinicians prefer verbal screening with informal questions such as "Do you worry often?" formal validated screening tools are often recommended. Examples of these include the Patient Health Questionnaire-9, Generalized Anxiety Disorder-7, Beck Depression Inventory, and Beck Anxiety Index. If screening indicates severe mood disorder, this should prompt further questioning and more urgent treatment. It is also important that clinicians have a clear strategy for dealing with a severely depressed or suicidal patient because depression and suicidality not uncommonly occur in headache or chronic pain patients. Any suicidal ideation should be taken seriously and immediately addressed. The patient should not be allowed to leave the office until thoroughly assessed by a physician. Obtain further history regarding plan or means to suicide (including access to firearms or lethal medications) as well as other risk factors for suicide (social isolation, substance abuse, etc.). If the patient is deemed to be a risk, they cannot be discharged from the office alone. Medical staff, emergency services, or law enforcement should accompany the patient to the nearest emergency department or mental health crises center. Suicide attempts seem to be more frequent in patients suffering from migraine than in the general population, especially in women and in those who have migraine with aura. Although cluster headache (CH) has been deemed the "suicide headache," reports of suicide in CH patients are rare and not well-evaluated.

Additional diagnostic testing should be considered on a case-by-case basis for headache patients endorsing psychiatric symptoms. Screening for thyroid disease, anemia, infectious processes, or vitamin deficiencies such as B_{12} or thiamine may be appropriate. In the patient presented here, screening for hypothyroidism would be appropriate given her recent weight gain, lethargy, and mood. A thorough medication reconciliation should be performed on every patient as well.

When treating headache patients, comorbid psychiatric conditions need to be taken into consideration. Attempts should be made to avoid headache medications that worsen mood. Cost, availability, and patient preference should also factor in. When psychiatric comorbidities are mild, monotherapy for prevention of migraine and mood can be considered. For example, in a patient who has mild anxiety, propranolol may be an appropriate choice for both migraine and symptoms of anxiety. In a patient who has insomnia and chronic migraine, a tricyclic antidepressant would be appropriate. Close monitoring of potential side effects and patient response to treatment is important. If a patient is not responding to monotherapy or if their psychiatric comorbidities are complex, using different treatment plans for each condition seems to improve outcomes. Medications used for both psychiatric conditions and headache are usually prescribed with different goal dosages and different titration plans. Collaboration with psychiatry on a treatment plan can ensure that both conditions are treated adequately and safely. If a patient is on several psychotropic medications, preventive options such as onabotulinumtoxinA, calcitonin gene-related peptide monoclonal antibodies, or neuromodulation should be considered.

In addition to medications, behavioral treatments should also be recommended. Mindfulness-based stress reduction, biofeedback, progressive muscle relaxation, and guided imagery coping skills are often used and helpful. In addition, cognitive-based strategies such as cognitive–behavioral therapy can be also utilized. The combination of medication and behavioral treatment has been found to be more effective than either medications or behavioral treatment alone.

KEY POINTS TO REMEMBER

- Screening for comorbid psychiatric disease is recommended in all headache patients because mood disorders increase the risk of development of headache chronicity, decrease quality of life, and complicate management.
- Suicide attempts seem to be more frequent in patients suffering from migraine than in the general population, especially in woman and those who have migraine with aura. It is important that clinicians have a clear strategy for dealing with a suicidal patient.
- Although monotherapy for mood disorder and migraine can be considered for mild cases, often a collaborative approach with psychiatry is necessary to ensure both psychiatric disease and headache are adequately managed.

Further Reading

Dresler T, Caratozzolo S, Guldolf K, et al. Understanding the nature of psychiatric comorbidity in migraine: A systematic review focused on interactions and treatment implications. *J Headache Pain*. 2019;20:51.

Heckman BD, Holroyd KA. Tension-type headache and psychiatric comorbidity. *Curr Pain Headache Rep*. 2006;10:439–447.

Minen MT, Begasse De Dhaem O, Kroon Van Diest A, et al. Migraine and its psychiatric comorbidities. *J Neurol Neurosurg Psychiatry*. 2016;87:741–749.

Robbins MS. The psychiatric comorbidities of cluster headache. *Curr Pain Headache Rep*. 2013;17:313.

A 48-year-old former alcoholic and heroin addict was involved in a motor vehicle accident 3 years prior. He was "T-boned" by a driver who ran a red light, and he subsequently experienced significant whiplash and hit his head on the window, resulting in transient loss of consciousness. Since the accident, he has experienced intractable daily headaches associated with photophobia, nausea, and difficulty concentrating. He endorses a history of prior migraine headaches; however, he states the intensity and frequency of his current headaches are worse. He has tried numerous treatment acute options, including ibuprofen, acetaminophen, sumatriptan, and naratriptan, to no avail. His primary care physician recently provided a limited prescription for hydrocodone given the patient states he is "desperate" and nothing else works. Magnetic resonance imaging without and with gadolinium done last year was negative. Exam is unremarkable.

What do you do now?

The most likely diagnosis here is persistent headache attributed to traumatic injury to the head. The patient also meets diagnostic criteria for chronic migraine. What complicates management, however, is the patient's prior history of substance abuse and his intractable nature to standard treatments.

Opioids have limited use in migraine, and the opioid epidemic is one of the greatest public health problems that the United States faces. Although there may be some benefit to adding them to other analgesic/abortive agents in very select cases of headache patients, regular use of opioids for headaches often leads to abuse and, at the very least, tolerance and increasing doses. Diverting opioids for the purpose of illicit selling for profit is an increasing problem as well.

When opioid use is considered reasonable and necessary, strict limits on amounts should be set. Patients should also sign an opioid medication contract that includes the agreement to undergo polydrug testing on a regular basis. Other key features of an opioid contract should include provisions to (1) prevent obtaining prescriptions for analgesics from more than one source, (2) ensure compliance with instructions about proper usage of medications, and (3) maintain a schedule of regular office visits. Contracts should also include details about consequences should any part of the agreement not be kept. Opioid contract samples are available at most institutions and on the internet, including the home pages of the American Academy for Pain Medicine (http://painmed.org) and the International Association for the Study of Pain (https://www.iasp-pain.org).

In patients with known prior substance abuse, opiates should always be avoided. In the presented case, there should be other options available. Options he may not have tried might include calcitonin gene-related peptide receptor antagonists or other nonsteroidal anti-inflammatories such as naproxen. Given headaches are daily, prophylactic treatment should be offered. Neuromodulation, nerve blockade, and behavioral strategies should be considered as well.

- Opioids are occasionally effective as adjunctive treatment in the setting of acute migraine, but their use as a regular abortive treatment is limited, particularly in cases in which there are medication addiction concerns.
- When using opioids or other drugs with addictive potential, strict medication limits, contracts, and drug testing are often indicated.

Further Reading

Arnold RM, Han PK, Seltzer D. Opioid contracts in chronic nonmalignant pain management: Objectives and uncertainties. *Am J Med*. 2006;119:292–296.

Coleman I, Rothney A, Wright SC, et al. Use of narcotic analgesics in the emergency department treatment of migraine headache. *Neurology*. 2004;62:1695–1700.

Koppin H, van Sonderen A, de Bruijn SFTM. Thunderclap headache. In: Ferrari A, Haan J, Charles A, Dodick DW, Sakai F, eds. *Oxford Textbook of Headache Syndromes*. Oxford, UK: Oxford University Press; 2020:307–313.

Questions Related to Special Populations

28 Menstrual Headaches

A 28-year-old woman has severe migraine headaches, particularly around menses. Some of her migraine attacks are preceded by visual aura symptoms, including scintillations and scotomata, that last at most 15 minutes. She develops photo- and phonophobia, but there are no other accompaniments. Headaches last at least 24 hours and can recur over several days. She also has severe menstrual cramps and typically experiences significant moodiness prior to her menstrual periods. Both migraine attacks and menstrual cramps have been dramatically reduced by an oral contraceptive containing both estrogen and progesterone. She is concerned about the safety of continuing this. Previous medications for migraine were ineffective except for zolmitriptan, which she uses effectively for the occasional migraine attacks that emerge.

What do you do now?

Menstrually related migraine (MRM) are typical during the time period this patient describes—from 2 days prior to the onset of menses, "d – 2," to the third day of flow, "d + 3." The majority of women with migraine, in fact, experience MRM. The headaches are generally not associated with auras, for unclear reasons. The two main proposed pathophysiological mechanisms of MRM are a drop in estrogen blood levels and prostaglandin release. It is likely that other mechanisms are yet to be identified. Many women report that their menstrual migraines are more severe, disabling, and refractory to treatment compared to migraines at other times of the month.

A different type of headache can occur premenstrually as part of the premenstrual syndrome (PMS) or premenstrual dysphoric disorder (PMDD), along with fatigue, emotional lability, anxiety, etc. These headaches generally have fewer migraine features and tend to respond to different treatment. Although there is some overlap between these two conditions, the patient described here seems to have MRM, as well as migraine with aura on occasion (probably nonmenstrually).

Triptans tend to be effective treatment for MRM and have even been used as "miniprophylaxis"—for example, orally on a bid schedule during the vulnerable times each month. Frovatriptan is particularly helpful when administered once daily as miniprophylaxis given its long half-life. Zolmitriptan also has good evidence for menstrual migraine, so it is not surprising that the patient responds to this. Nonsteroidal anti-inflammatory drugs (NSAIDs), particularly naproxen and mefenamic acid, have also been shown to be of benefit. It is likely that her estrogen–progesterone oral contraceptive (EPOC) is helping both her MRM and menstrual cramps because both conditions can be improved in this way for many women. The severe menstrual cramps she experiences may in fact be a clue that she has endometriosis, a condition comorbid with migraine and responsive to hormonal treatment. This might be worth investigation by her gynecologist.

The problem here lies with the accepted belief that estrogen-containing medications should be avoided in patients with migraine with aura. Data strongly suggest that both migraine and oral contraceptives are associated with an increased risk of ischemic stroke, and patients with migraine with aura have a greater risk than women with migraine without aura (for a review, see McGregor, 2013). Interestingly, there are no compelling data concerning the stroke risk for older women using hormone replacement therapy. It will be important to see what this patient's headache log reveals—how frequent the headaches are, how often she experiences aura, how long it lasts, and whether any of her menstrual headaches are accompanied by aura. One suspects that virtually all of her menstrual migraines are sans aura.

So, what to do here? A good first step is always to discuss tough decisions such as this with the patient. She is reluctant to make a change and for good reason—things are going well. When she understands the stroke risk, she will likely agree to try alternatives because there are some good ones. Initially, discontinuing the EPOC and seeing her gynecologist about contraceptive options, PMS, and menstrual cramps would be reasonable. Trying triptan miniprophylaxis—that is, daily during the vulnerable d − 2 through d + 3 or beyond—might be very effective, sticking with the triptan she is comfortable with. If this does not work, then NSAIDs in combination with PRN triptan use might work or perhaps institution of a prophylactic agent such as topiramate, a beta-blocker, or a cyclic antidepressant might be appropriate, particularly if the headache log reveals a high frequency. (However, if the treatment for this patient's PMS ends up being a selective serotonin reuptake inhibitor, the most useful class of medication for PMDD, a cyclic antidepressant may not be the best choice.) If the choice is made to use anticonvulsant medication, it is important to warn the patient that any of these may reduce the contraceptive effectiveness of the oral contraceptive pill. If this does not work out, phytoestrogens (e.g., genistein and daidzein) might help the symptoms that her EPOC helped. There is not much evidence yet for this, but it seems to offer benefit to some women. Magnesium at high dose either perimenstrually or continuously at a dosage of 500–600 mg daily has also been effective for some women with MRM (see Table 28.1 for a list of preventive treatment options in MRM).

However, if the previously mentioned approaches fail and this patient wants to return to hormonal treatment, it is not irresponsible to consider this as an option, considering the fact that the stroke risk in her age group, even with migraine with aura and estrogen intake, is quite low if there are no other risk factors such as tobacco use, hypertension, hyperlipidemia, obesity, or diabetes. Trying a progesterone-only agent is unlikely to help

TABLE 28.1 **Preventive Treatment of Menstrual Migraine**

Medication Class	Examples	Dose
Triptans	Zolmitriptan	2.5 mg bid–tid d – 3–d + 4
	Naratriptan po	1–2.5 mg bid d – 3–d + 4
	Frovatriptan po	2.5 mg once daily d – 3–d + 4
NSAIDs	Naproxen sodium	550 mg bid d – 3–d + 4
	Mefanamic acid	500 mg bid d – 3–d + 4
Beta-blockers	Atenolol	25 mg bid or d – 3–d + 4
	Metoprolol	50 mg daily or d – 3–d + 4
Magnesium	Magnesium gluconate	500–600 mg daily
Estrogen	Estrogen + progesterone combination medication	Extended-cycle regimen (typical for oral contraceptive pills)
	Estrogen alone—oral, transdermal	d – 3–d + 4 or 3-month courses
Phytoestrogens	Soy extract	Daily or d – 3–d + 4

NSAIDs, nonsteroidal anti-inflammatory drugs.

migraines and, in fact, might exacerbate them. One could return to an EPOC, although the lowest dose possible would be optimal. Constant daily use of EPOC, as an extended cycle regimen, is a commonly used strategy to prevent menstrually related attacks. However, EPOC is not consistently helpful; migraine can become worse (in approximately 25%), stay the same (in approximately 50%), or become less frequent (in approximately 25%). Hysterectomy and oophorectomy are often necessary in women for many reasons, but they should never be implemented with the sole purpose of lessening migraine. Women with migraine who are thrown into menopause afterwards frequently experience worsening. Of the calcitonin gene-related peptide antagonists, monoclonal antibodies, and ditans now available, current data on efficacy for menstrual migraine are lacking, but they may play a beneficial role once additional data is available.

- Menstrual migraine is a common form of migraine, generally presenting as migraine without aura, and can be more severe and disabling than migraine attacks at other times of the month.
- Focused miniprophylaxis treatments during the perimenstrual period can be very successful, but acute treatments are generally necessary as well, including triptans.
- Estrogenic agents are contraindicated in younger women who have migraine with aura because of postulated increased stroke risks, although their use can sometimes be justified if low doses are used and other risk factors are minimized.

Further Reading

Burch R. Epidemiology and treatment of menstrual migraine and migraine during pregnancy and lactation: A narrative review. *Headache.* 2020;60:200–216.

Burke BE, Olson RD, Cusack BJ. Randomized, controlled trial of phytoestrogen in the prophylactic treatment of menstrual migraine. *Biomed Pharmacother.* 2002;56:283–288.

McGregor EA. Contraception and headache. *Headache.* 2013;53:247–276.

Tzourio C, Tehindrazanarivelo A, Iglésias S, et al. Case–control study of migraine and risk of ischaemic stroke in young women. *BMJ.* 1995;310:830–833.

Vetvik K, MacGregor EA. Menstrual migraine: A distinct disorder needing greater recognition. *Lancet Neurol.* 2021;20:304–315.

29 Headaches in Pregnancy

A 21-week pregnant mother of two describes a long history of menstrual and occasionally nonmenstrual migrainous headaches. For the past 6 weeks, however, she has noted a significant exacerbation of headaches to a near daily frequency, often accompanied by significant nausea with some vomiting. Although she has not had auras before, she has recently had some visual changes, including blurred vision and scintillating lights in her peripheral visual fields around the time of headaches. The nausea has led to a 5-pound weight loss during the past month. Her examination is normal, although her affect seems depressed and she looks tired. She is taking only prenatal vitamins.

What do you do now?

Most women with migraine experience improvement, and even remission, in their headaches during pregnancy by the time of their second trimester. This seems to be even more likely in women with menstrually related migraine. But there are still many women who experience the opposite trend with, at times, disabling pain and nausea. Auras can occur for the first time during pregnancy as well. The first medical decision is how seriously to work up the changes in her migraine symptoms (increased frequency and aura). Gestational hypertension and preeclampsia must be ruled out. Migraine appears to be a risk factor for preeclampsia, and there is evidence that eclampsia occurs earlier in women with migraine. Hypertension can lead to the posterior reversible encephalopathy syndrome, which can present with headache but also generally includes focal neurological signs. Without focal neurological deficits, an intracranial mass or infectious process is unlikely. Pituitary hemorrhage is less likely during the second trimester but can occur. Reversible cerebral vasoconstriction syndrome was termed "postpartum angiopathy" due to its predilection for pregnancy and postpartum periods, and it may present with only headaches, often of sudden onset ("thunderclap"; (see Chapter 14). Cerebral venous thrombosis, cervical arterial dissection (see Chapter 5), and idiopathic intracranial hypertension (also known as pseudotumor cerebri) (see Chapter 22) are also possible explanations for new or intensification of prior headaches in pregnancy. So, if there is any suspicion or if there are even subtle neurological findings on exam, a head magnetic resonance imaging, magnetic resonance venogram, and lumbar puncture would be mandatory.

Once secondary headache causes have been eliminated, migraine treatment during pregnancy generally begins with a concerted effort to pursue nonpharmacological measures. Most texts emphasize the importance of reassurance and stressing the high chance of improvement by the third trimester and following delivery. But this is of small comfort to patients such as this one, and there is the real possibility that ongoing severe migraines may themselves lead to fetal compromise, particularly if there is vomiting and dehydration.

Manual therapy including cervical massage and acupressure may be of help for migraine in pregnancy, and muscle relaxation with or without biofeedback training can also be useful. Formerly, magnesium supplementation was often found to be an effective treatment of migraine during pregnancy, but recent concerns about its interference with fetal calcium metabolism have discouraged its use. Riboflavin is probably safe and may help at a dose of 400 mg daily.

Medication choices in pregnancy are limited. There are some data concerning drug safety in pregnancy, but sources of information differ. The U.S. Food and Drug Administration (FDA) provided a listing of relative safety using five categories—A–D and X (Box 29.1)—although it has recently abandoned this rating system. Unfortunately, very few drugs were in the "safer" categories (A and B), and many drugs were not rated. Another rating system, the Teratogen Information Service, also provided risk categories for many drugs from "no risk" to "high." Unfortunately, many drugs were rated "undetermined" or "unlikely."

Acetaminophen is in FDA category B and is useful for acute headache management for some patients. The use of opioids (e.g., codeine, hydrocodone, oxycodone, and morphine) during pregnancy is controversial. The only opioids that are category B are oxycodone, butorphanol, and meperidine, but meperidine's metabolite, normeperidine, is particularly long-lived and can lead to toxicity, including a lowering of seizure threshold in susceptible patients. Ibuprofen and naproxen sodium, both effective as acute treatment for many migraine patients, are FDA category C but become category D in the third trimester because nonsteroidal

---

BOX 29.1 **FDA Pregnancy Risk Categories**

Category A: Controlled human studies indicate no apparent risk to fetus. The possibility of harm to the fetus appears remote.

Category B: Either animal studies do not indicate a fetal risk or animal studies do indicate a teratogenic risk, but well-controlled human studies have failed to demonstrate the same risk.

Category C: Studies indicate teratogenic or embryocidal risks in animals, but no controlled studies have been done in women, or there are no controlled studies in animals or humans.

Category D: Positive evidence of human fetal risk, but in certain circumstances, the benefits of the drug may outweigh the risk involved.

Category X: Positive evidence of significant fetal risk, and the risk clearly outweighs any possible benefit.

anti-inflammatory drugs (NSAIDs) can interfere with closure of the ductus arteriosus. They also may lead to bleeding complications if used around the time of delivery. Aspirin is a category C drug in the first two trimesters but changes to category D if given in the third trimester (for the same reasons as those for NSAIDs). Caffeine is also category C. Triptans, particularly sumatriptan, seem to be safe during pregnancy, with mounting evidence to support their use, but all have remained in category C. Prednisone and methylprednisolone were placed in category C but are quite effective in breaking a cycle of headache and might be considered. (Dexamethasone is category D). Ergots, including ergotamine and dihydroergotamine, are category X due to their effects on implantation of the embryo, uterine blood flow, and fetal development, as well as their tendency to produce uterine contractions (Table 29.1).

Of the antiemetics, metoclopramide is in category B and is useful not only for nausea but also for antimigraine effects of its own and its possible promotion of the absorption of other analgesics. The phenothiazine antiemetics such as prochlorperazine and promethazine are in category C, but they are used when nausea and vomiting lead to dehydration and/or metabolic imbalances in pregnant women. Ondansetron is category B, but there has been some concern about cleft palate. Emetrol (phosphorylated cola syrup), although relatively weak, can be of use with nausea as well.

TABLE 29.1 **Selected Acute and Prophylactic Migraine Medications Considered Reasonably Safe for Use in Pregnancy[1]**

Acute Headache Treatment	Antiemetic	Prophylactic Interventions
Acetaminophen	Ondansetron	Riboflavin
Ibuprofen, naproxen	Metoclopramide	Memantine
Oxycodone	Promethazine	Cyproheptadine
Sumatriptan	Ginger	Lidocaine, ropivicaine[2]

[1]All interventions for treatment of migraine in pregnancy must be first discussed with obstetric specialists, as data arises regularly.
[2]For nerve blocks.

Ginger in the form of candied ginger or encapsulated desiccated ginger can be very helpful (see Table 29.1).

Prophylactic agents such as beta blockers, calcium channel blockers and cyclic antidepressants are all category C agents (except for atenolol which is category D) and may not be particularly effective at preventing migraine during pregnancy. Depakote and Topiramate are in category D due to teratogenicity. Memantine is category B and might be a useful prophylactic medication in our patient once secondary causes are set aside; dose is in the 5–20 mg per day range in two divided doses. Another category B medication cyproheptadine, can also be useful in selected cases in the dose of a 4-8 mg daily (Table 29.1). A number of medications used to treat migraine can alter folate metabolism so precautionary supplementation with 400 mcg folate daily is advisable when using daily medications.

Temporary blockade of greater and lesser occipital nerves has anecdotally been very useful in pregnancy. Lidocaine and ropivicaine (category B) are preferred over bupivacaine (category C). Myofascial trigger point injections of these local anesthetics in pericranial and cervical muscle groups can be of help as well. Botulinum toxin probably does not pass through the placenta because of its molecular size, but risks are not fully known. Neurostimulation devices are probably safe in pregnancy, particularly forms of transcutaneous nerve stimulation such as the supraorbital stimulator device Cefaly®. Transcutaneous vagal nerve stimulation and transcranial magnetic stimulation for acute and preventive migraine treatment should be safe, but this is not yet certain. It is important to remember, of course, that before starting any of the treatment options discussed, it is wise for pregnant patients to consult with their obstetric and pediatric team regarding their safety.

In the current case, a number of factors suggest an aggressive approach to headaches, including high headache frequency and severity, nausea and vomiting, weight loss, and depression. Diagnostic evaluation should be done, guided by careful neurological examinations. Antinauseant medication should be employed, and acute and perhaps preventive treatment should be instituted. Occipital nerve blocks, manual therapy, and muscle relaxation training might prove very useful. A detailed empathetic discussion of risks and benefits should allay the patient's fears and promote hopefulness.

- Although migraines improve during pregnancy for most women, there are many cases of the opposite, sometimes accompanied by severe nausea and vomiting.
- Diagnostic suspicion should be high with any change in headache pattern, although most headaches will be benign.
- Nonpharmacological therapy can help migraines in pregnancy, but judicious supplementation with pharmaceutical treatments is reasonable, particularly in severe cases.

Further Reading

Briggs, GB, Freeman, RK, Towers, CV, Forinash, AB. *Drugs in Pregnancy and Lactation: A Reference Guide to Fetal and Neonatal Risk*. 11th ed. Philadelphia, PA: Lippincott Williams & Wilkins; 2017.

Jemel M, Kandara H, Riahi M, Gharbi R, Nagi S, Kamoun I. Gestational pituitary apoplexy: Case series and review of the literature. *J Gynecol Obstet Hum Reprod*. 2019;48:873–881.

Negro A, Delaruelle Z, Ivanova TA, et al. Headache and pregnancy: A systematic review. *J Headache Pain*. 2017;18:106.

Robbins MS. Headache in pregnancy. *CONTINUUM*. 2018;24:1092–1107.

Sandoe CH, Lay C. Secondary headaches during pregnancy: When to worry. *Curr Neurol Neurosci Rep*. 2019;19:27.

Spielmann K, Kayser A, Beck E, Meister R, Schaefer C. Pregnancy outcome after anti-migraine triptan use: A prospective observational cohort study. *Cephalalgia*. 2018;38:1081–1092.

30 Combined Hormonal Contraceptives and Migraine

Specialties: Neurology, Primary Care, Obstetrics and Gynecology

A 19-year-old woman with polycystic ovarian syndrome (PCOS) was referred by her internist to discuss contraception options, given that she also has migraine. She has no other health issues and is a nonsmoker. Her only medications are metformin 500 mg daily for PCOS; sumatriptan 100 mg for the acute treatment of migraine, which she needs to use approximately three or four times a month; and naproxen 440 mg as needed for menstrual pain. Upon further discussion, she explains that she consistently will have a migraine attack the day her menstrual cycle begins each month, and this attack is generally more debilitating and frequently refractory to sumatriptan. Outside of the menstrual window, she typically has two or three additional migraine attacks each month, and these attacks sometimes begin with a visual aura of jagged bright lines lasting 20 minutes prior to the headache onset. Her menstrual cycles are often heavy, painful, and irregular, and she is interested in trying combined hormonal contraception to see if that will help. Her internist has requested neurological clearance before starting any estrogen-containing contraceptives.

What do you do now?

There are several things to consider. A diagnosis of aura has been established as a stroke risk factor and can double a woman's baseline stroke risk; this risk can increase further if aura occurs frequently. Although there is no contraindication in using combined hormonal contraceptives (CHCs) in women who have migraine without aura, they have been contraindicated in women who have aura due to concern of increasing ischemic stroke risk even further. However, this risk is based on data from the 1960s and 1970s, when estrogen doses in CHCs were commonly 150 μg, which is significantly higher than current options. Today's CHCs typically contain estrogen at doses of 30 μg or less, and these low doses do not lead to the same sort of stroke risk. Ischemic stroke risk with CHCs is dependent on the dose of estrogen. Doses of 20 μg or less do not increase stroke risk in healthy women who do not smoke.

Estrogen impacts migraine in different ways. High levels of estrogen can trigger aura. This fact explains why when new-onset migraine occurs during pregnancy, it is more likely to be migraine with aura given the higher levels of estrogen present. Sudden drops in estrogen, such as during menses, can also trigger migraine in women who have this hormonal link. Consequently, during puberty and perimenopause, when menstrual irregularity is more likely to be present, women often experience worsening of migraine attacks. Thus, current data suggest that using a CHC formulation that contains no more than 20 μg of estrogen on a continuous basis may help prevent migraine and may also reduce the risk of stroke by preventing estrogen fluctuations and reducing aura frequency.

Using CHCs to not only help treat menstrually related migraine but also help prevent aura and reduce stroke risk is a relatively new idea, and it signals that we may be in the midst of a paradigm shift in the way we think about hormones and migraine.

A 2010 practice bulletin from the American College of Obstetrics and Gynecology acknowledged that using continuous or extended-cycle CHCs can help prevent menstrually related migraine, but it cautioned against using estrogen-containing contraceptives in women with focal neurologic signs (including aura), women who smoke, and women older than age 35 years. The authors of the practice bulletin reasoned that although stroke is rare, the impact of a stroke can be devastating, and other contraception options that do not include estrogen are available with less risk. A 2017 consensus statement from the European Headache Federation and the European Society of Contraception and Reproductive Health, based on a systematic review of the existing literature, identified that we lack robust data on risks of CHCs in women with aura and that more research is needed to help guide clinical decision-making. Given the current landscape, both of these statements highlight the need to carefully consider the particular needs and situation of the individual patient and take these into account when making recommendations.

Because aura is considered a stroke risk factor, and because there remains controversy regarding whether or not women with aura can use estrogen-containing contraceptives, it is extremely important to be aware of what is and what is not aura and to give patients the most accurate diagnosis possible. According to the *International Classification of Headache Disorders*, third edition, aura is a positive focal symptom or symptoms, spreading gradually over 5 minutes, lasting 5–60 minutes, and often followed by a headache within 60 minutes. Visual aura is the most common. With that in mind, when patients mention they have visual blurring, split-second visual flashes, or momentary floaters in their vision, these are not aura. Asking detailed questions and taking a careful history is crucial.

Ultimately, as we await further clinical data and consensus across the various organizations that are stakeholders in women's health, we can use the existing data to help counsel patients on risks and benefits to help them make the most informed decision possible. The patient in this case is young, a nonsmoker, and does not have any other medical issues including any coagulopathies or other stroke risk factors beyond migraine with aura. If her only goal was to prevent pregnancy, we could recommend using a non-estrogen approach because there are several such options available. However, estrogen therapy does have benefits beyond contraception, and given her history of both migraine with aura and menstrually related migraine, trialing a low-dose continuous or extended-cycle CHC is reasonable. If she chooses that route, following up in a few months to assess aura and menstrually related migraine improvement would be important. We can tailor our recommendations to the needs of the individual patient.

- Women who have migraine without aura can use CHCs without any restrictions.
- There is debate on the use of estrogen-containing contraceptives in women who have migraine with aura.
- Although aura is associated with a twofold increase in stroke risk, it is important to note that the absolute risk of stroke remains small in young healthy women who do not smoke.
- Be aware of the definition of aura and that split-second visual disturbances or visual blurring are not aura.

Further Reading

Calhoun AH, Batur P. Combined hormonal contraceptives and migraine: An update on the evidence. *Cleve Clin J Med.* 2017;84(8):631–638.

Gryglas A, Smigiel R. Migraine and stroke: What's the link? What to do? *Curr Neurol Neurosci Rep.* 2017;17(3):22.

Sacco S, Merki-Feld GS, Ægidius KL, et al.; European Headache Federation and the European Society of Contraception and Reproductive Health. Effect of exogenous estrogens and progestogens on the course of migraine during reproductive age: A consensus statement by the European Headache Federation (EHF) and the European Society of Contraception and Reproductive Health (ESCRH). *J Headache Pain.* 2018;19(1):76. doi:10.1186/s10194-018-0896-5

Sheikh HU, Pavlovic J, Loder E, Burch R. Risk of stroke associated with use of estrogen containing contraceptives in women with migraine: A systematic review. *Headache.* 2018;58(1):5–21.

Voedisch AJ, Hindiyeh N. Combined hormonal contraception and migraine: Are we being too strict? *Curr Opin Obstet Gynecol.* 2019;31(6):452–458.

31 Abdominal Migraine

An 8-year-old boy presents to the emergency department (ED) with severe abdominal pain for the past 24–36 hours. This pain is periumbilical and associated with nausea and pallor. He had one episode of vomiting today and has been unable to keep much down given discomfort and nausea. He denies any other associated symptoms. His mother states this has occurred a few other times in the past year; however, his prior episodes typically resolved within 4–6 hours and were not as severe. He is an otherwise normal and healthy young boy, but his mother does say he was "colicky" when he was young. On exam, he is afebrile, and vitals are otherwise stable. His abdomen is nondistended, and bowel sounds are normal. He is mildly tender to touch, but no guarding or rebound tenderness are present. In the ED, basic labs and computed tomography of the abdomen are performed and are normal. On further history, his mother endorses that she personally has a history of migraine. The family is otherwise healthy

What do you do now?

Given this patient has already had a fairly thorough exam and workup, one must be reassured that insidious gastrointestinal diseases such as appendicitis or bowel obstruction are ruled out. Given his family history of migraine in his mother and personal history of infantile colic, it is most likely that he is experiencing abdominal migraine.

Abdominal migraine is classified as an episodic syndrome that may be associated with migraine although headache is absent. This syndrome typically affects children aged 3–12 years. Another episodic syndrome that causes recurrent gastrointestinal disturbance is cyclical vomiting syndrome. These syndromes describe periodic symptoms in children who commonly have a family history of migraine, have co-occurrence of migraine, or have an increased risk of clinical evolution to migraine in later years. Abdominal migraine has been reported in adults; however, it is believed to be much less common. Infantile colic has also been suggested as another episodic syndrome potentially linked to migraine.

Abdominal migraine affects girls more often than boys and is the most common episodic syndrome to present to pediatric headache clinics. The diagnosis of abdominal migraine is made clinically and outlined in Box 31.1. There can be a premonitory phase of behavioral irritability. Attacks often interfere with functioning, and headache is not present during episodes. If headache is present, one should consider the diagnosis of

---

BOX 31.1   **ICHD-3 Diagnostic Criteria for Abdominal Migraine**

A. At least five attacks of abdominal pain, fulfilling criteria B–D
B. Pain has at least two of the following three characteristics:
   1. Midline location, periumbilical or poorly localized
   2. Dull or "just sore" quality
   3. Moderate or severe intensity
C. At least two of the following four associated symptoms or signs:
   1. Anorexia
   2. Nausea
   3. Vomiting
   4. Pallor
D. Attacks last 2–72 hours when untreated or unsuccessfully treated
E. Complete freedom from symptoms between attacks
F. Not attributed to another disorder

ICHD-3, *International Classification of Headache Disorders*, third edition.

migraine without aura. In contrast to cyclical vomiting syndrome (see clinical criteria in Box 31.2), the vomiting in abdominal migraine is often less prominent. Constipation and/or diarrhea is generally not present in abdominal migraine and can be a helpful differentiating characteristic to irritable bowel syndrome. In addition, it is important that the attacks are not associated with illness, fever, or evidence of metabolic disease. If all red flags are excluded, no further investigation is necessary.

With regard to management of abdominal migraine, the most important first step is proper diagnosis and education. Lifestyle modification can be very helpful, including maintaining a regular schedule, sleep hygiene, and adequate nutrition. Behavioral treatments that are helpful in migraine, such as cognitive–behavioral therapy, should be considered as well.

The pharmacological options for abdominal migraine are similar to those for cyclical vomiting syndrome. Preventively, several retrospective studies have shown promise for propranolol, cyproheptadine, amitriptyline, and topiramate. Acutely, one can consider strategies extrapolated from acute treatment of pediatric migraine, such as triptans and over-the-counter analgesics, because specific acute treatments for abdominal migraine do not exist. Case studies have supported the use of acute nasal sumatriptan or intravenous dihydroergotamine. Antiemetics should be considered as well. See Table 31.1 for dosing. It is unknown if newer migraine-specific therapies such as anti–calcitonin gene-related peptide monoclonal antibodies will be efficacious in treating the episodic syndromes of childhood.

TABLE 31.1 **Treatment of Abdominal Migraine**

General	Explanation and education of patient and family (avoid triggers, regular lifestyle, behavioral treatments such as cognitive–behavioral therapy)
Acute	Rest in a dark, quiet room
	Simple analgesics such as paracetamol 15 mg/kg, ibuprofen 10 mg/kg
	Sumatriptan 10 mg intranasal
	Intravenous dihydroergotamine 0.5 mg/dose
Preventive	Propranolol 2–4 mg/kg/day up to 10–20 mg bid or tid
	Cyproheptadine 0.25 mg/kg/day up to 8 mg at bedtime
	Topiramate 5–9 mg/kg/day up to 100 mg/day
	Valproic acid 10–40 mg/kg/day
	Amitriptyline 0.5–1 mg/kg/day at bedtime

KEY POINTS TO REMEMBER

- Abdominal migraine is a poorly understood episodic syndrome of childhood affecting children aged 3–12 years. Abdominal migraine is not associated with headache; however, it has a propensity to develop into migraine in later years.
- Diagnosis is made clinically; however, if any red flags are raised—including failure to thrive, unexplained or recurrent fevers, chronic diarrhea, anemia, or family history of inflammatory bowel disease—concern should be raised for an alternative diagnosis and diagnostic evaluation should ensue.
- Treatment strategies are often extrapolated from migraine treatment and should include both pharmacological and nonpharmacological options.

Further Reading

Angus-Leppan H. Abdominal migraine. *BMJ*. 2018;360:k179.

Billinghurst L, Richer L, Russell K, et al. Systematic review of acute migraine therapy in children. *Headache*. 2004;44:464–465.

Irwin S, Barmherzig R, Gelfand A. Recurrent gastrointestinal disturbance: Abdominal migraine and cyclical vomiting syndrome. *Curr Neurol Neurosci Rep*. 2017;17:21.

Napthali K, Koloski N, Talley NJ. Abdominal migraine. *Cephalalgia*. 2016;36(10):980–986.

32 Acute Treatment of Childhood Migraine

An 11-year-old, 28-kg girl has had severe unilateral throbbing headaches for the past 2 years. They are accompanied by nausea and vomiting, photophobia, phonophobia, and fatigue. Headaches occur approximately once per month but can occur more frequently during hot weather and with stress (e.g., around the time her parents were contemplating divorce). Her headaches are dramatically responsive to zolmitriptan 5 mg, although she experiences a 20-minute period of very bothersome aching pain and tension in her jaw and neck. She is now out of zolmitriptan.

What do you do now?

This child almost certainly has migraine. The diagnosis of migraine in children is slightly challenging because the features may differ from the standard definition in adults. Specifically, the headaches may be shorter, they are commonly bilateral, and auras are rarer. Treatment has typically centered around nonpharmacological measures such as sleep hygiene, regular mealtimes, and avoidance of triggers, with the judicious use of analgesics and antiemetics. However, this is not a satisfying approach when the child has very severe headaches that are disabling. Participation in school, social, and family activities will be affected, and the child can develop secondary psychological consequences. Both acute treatment of headaches and prophylaxis should be planned concurrently. A number of prophylactic agents are in common use, although few have a formal U.S. Food and Drug Administration (FDA) indication for prevention of migraine in children. Beta-blockers, cyclic antidepressants, calcium channel blockers, and the anticonvulsants divalproex sodium (Depakote) and topiramate (Topamax) have been shown to help some children and adolescents. Cyproheptadine (Periactin) has been advocated for some time as a useful preventive agent as well. These medications have the potential to affect (to varying degrees) energy levels, sleep patterns, and cognition, so careful monitoring of adverse effects must be a high priority. Parents are often quite interested in the use of substances other than medications for treatment. Many vitamins, minerals, and supplements are often considered. Riboflavin, melatonin, and magnesium in particular should be considered. Emerging therapies such as neurostimulation and calcitonin gene-related peptide (CGRP) monoclonal antibodies are promising; however, there is a paucity of data in children.

In the analgesic class, ibuprofen and acetaminophen have the best evidence supporting their use in children. Other nonsteroidal anti-inflammatory drugs (NSAIDs), such as naproxen sodium, have been widely used as well. Antiemetics such as promethazine (Phenergan) and metoclopramide (Reglan) can be very effective when used judiciously. Extrapyramidal symptoms related to antiemetic/neuroleptic medication use, including akathisia (restlessness) and dystonia (muscular spasms of the neck, eyes, tongue, or jaw), are more common in children than adults, so close observation is indicated.

If a child's migraine attacks are not responsive to analgesics, a triptan is indicated. Only rizatriptan (orally disintegrating tablet) has gained FDA approval for use in children (ages 6 years or older). Almotriptan (po), zolmitriptan (nasal), and sumatriptan/naproxen (po) have FDA approval for use in adolescents (ages 12 years or older). The majority of triptan contraindications are rare in pediatric patients because children tend to be healthy from a vascular standpoint. Serious triptan complications related to hypertension and vascular constriction seem to be virtually nonexistent. Children do experience the less serious, but still troublesome, adverse effects seen in the general population, such as jaw tightness and other muscular symptoms, sensation changes, sedation, and nausea. They may also experience central nervous system side effects, which can interfere with school performance. One of the features of the triptans most written about is the fact that their effects differ among users. This is sometimes so marked as to prompt the trial of multiple triptans in patients to find the most effective and least offensive agent (Box 32.1).

In this case, two steps should be taken. First, the safety of triptans should not be taken entirely for granted. A thorough physical exam should be given to ensure cardiovascular and other systems are normal. Because the features of this girl's headaches are so suggestive of migraine, neuroimaging is probably not essential, particularly if there is a strong family history. Of course, full neurological and head and neck exams must be done, and diagnostic decision-making should always be discussed fully with the parents. Second, if no contraindications are found to the use of triptans, an alternative triptan might be tried in the hope of avoiding the annoying jaw and neck tightness (Table 32.1). Perhaps rizatriptan or almotriptan could be tried because these seem to have fewer adverse effects. Doses are not clearly known, but half of the usual adult dose would seem reasonable given this patient's weight.

BOX 32.1 **Common Triptan Side Effects**

Dizziness, lightheadedness
Paresthesias, hot or cold sensations
Nausea
Muscular pain and tightness
Dry mouth
Chest pain (generally noncardiac)

TABLE 32.1 **Acute Medications Used in Treating Migraine in Children**[1]

Medication	Typical Dose
Ibuprofen	200–800 mg or 5–10 mg/kg
Acetaminophen	325–650 mg or 10 mg/kg
Acetaminophen with codeine	300 mg + 30 mg po
Sumatriptan	25–50 mg po or 5 mg nasal
Almotriptan	6.5 mg po
Zolmitriptan	2.5 mg po
Rizatriptan	5 mg po
Naratriptan	1.25–2.5 mg po
Eletriptan	20–40 mg po
Promethazine (Phenergan)	12.5 mg suppository, 25 mg po (for nausea)
Metoclopramide (Reglan)	5 mg po (for nausea)

[1]Typical doses for children >40 kg are shown, although evidence for effectiveness and tolerance is incomplete.

Another thought is to try an NSAID or acetaminophen in combination with a triptan. Melatonin has been studied for acute treatment in pediatric migraine with positive results and therefore can also be considered. Neuromodulation devices are often utilized for acute treatment and may even be favorable in the pediatric population given the low side effect profile. If deemed appropriate, the novel CGRP receptor antagonists ubrogepant and rimegepant, although not studied yet in the pediatric population, are probably also an option given their favorable side effect profile and safety.

KEY POINTS TO REMEMBER

- Migraine in children differs from the adult form in several ways: (1) The headache can be shorter; (2) unilaterality is less common; and (3) auras are less common.
- Lifestyle adjustment can be very helpful in pediatric migraine.

- Although only rizatriptan (Maxalt) is approved for use in children, judicious use of triptans with open discussion with parents is common practice. Novel treatment modalities such as melatonin, neuromodulation, and CGRP receptor antagonists should be considered as well.
- Both acute medications and prophylactic agents may produce significant adverse effects in children that must be monitored closely.

Further Reading

Gelfand AA, Ross AC, Irwin SL, Greene KA, Qubty WF, Allen E. Melatonin for acute treatment of migraine in children and adolescents: A pilot randomized trial. *Headache*. 2020;60:1712–1721.

Gladstein J. Triptans in children and adolescents. *Drug Dev Res.* 2007;68:346–349.

O'Brien HL, Kabbouche MA, Hershey AD. Treating pediatric migraine: An expert opinion. *Expert Opin Pharmacother.* 2012;13(7):959–966.

Patniyot IR, Gelfand AA. Acute treatment therapies for pediatric migraine: A qualitative systematic review. *Headache*. 2016;56:49–70.

33 Chronic Headache in an Adolescent

A 17-year old girl accompanied by her parents presents for her first visit. She reports developing migraines without aura at age 11 years that were infrequent and easily treated with over-the-counter medications. Attacks increased to five to seven times monthly at age 14 years, and for the past year they have occurred at least 15 days per month. Headaches can be left- or right-sided, throbbing, moderate to severe in intensity, and associated with nausea, photophobia, and phonophobia. She has been treated with appropriate doses for at least 3 months of riboflavin, magnesium, cyproheptadine, propranolol, topiramate, valproic acid, verapamil, and amitriptyline without benefit or with intolerable side effects. Currently, she is taking nortriptyline 50 mg nightly and sees a psychologist for biofeedback and cognitive–behavioral therapy (CBT). She uses almotriptan twice weekly with good results; however, on other days, she avoids acute medications and tries to "ride it out." She and her parents are concerned that although she has never missed school, she is finding it more difficult to keep up with her work and worries she will not be able to attend college next year. They ask if there are any newer preventive agents available for her.

What do you do now?

M igraine affects approximately 20% of adolescents, and chronic migraine (≥15 headache days per month with at least 8 of those meeting criteria for migraine for more than 3 months) affects up to 1.8% of them. Chronic migraine is disabling and has a significant impact on the adolescent's self-esteem, quality of life (QOL), family and social functioning, and scholastic success. Yet, chronic migraine in this age group remains underdiagnosed, undertreated, and inadequately studied. In fact, since the initial pharmacologic treatment guidelines were developed in 2004, only 21 additional studies met the criteria for inclusion.

The goals of migraine prevention are primarily to reduce the frequency and severity of individual attacks and to improve QOL. Typically, preventive treatments are initiated when attacks occur 4 or more days monthly or when migraine is disabling or negatively impacts QOL. Several tools are available to measure the impact of migraine in this age group and to help guide treatment options. Two useful tools in clinical practice are PedMIDAS to measure disability and PedsQL to measure health-related QOL. Prevention should be given when PedMIDAS scores are high (>30) or when PedsQL scores are low.

In general, choosing migraine prevention is often based on the presence or absence of other comorbidities or co-occurring conditions. Migraine prevention encompasses lifestyle modifications and nonpharmacologic and pharmacological therapies. These modalities may be used together. Lifestyle modifications include regular sleep patterns, eating habits, exercise routines, hydration, and stress reduction. The patient, parents, and often school personnel need to be involved to ensure success.

Patients who experience high-frequency or chronic migraine often overuse acute medications. Medication overuse is not only a risk factor for migraine chronification but also a reason for preventive medication failure, and as such identification and elimination of medication overuse are paramount to ensure the best possible outcome.

Currently, only one preventive therapy (topiramate) is specifically approved for the prevention of migraine in adolescents, yet several are often used off-label. Amitriptyline and nortriptyline are commonly employed as migraine prevention in this age group, in doses ranging from 10 to 75 mg daily. They are usually initiated at a 10- to 25-mg bedtime dose and gradually increased every 4–6 weeks. Common side effects include sedation, dry mouth, blurry vision, constipation, and weight gain. Electrocardiogram monitoring should be done at doses greater than 40 mg to identify prolonged QRS or Q-T intervals. The U.S. Food and Drug Administration (FDA) issued a black box warning for the use of all antidepressants in children and adolescents because of the risk of suicidal behavior. The beta-blocker propranolol, although approved for adults with migraine, and often used in this age group, has not demonstrated efficacy in clinical trials of adolescents. Doses range from 80 to 240 mg daily.

The anti-epileptic medications sodium valproate and topiramate have been studied in pediatric and adolescent migraine, and as mentioned previously, topiramate is FDA approved for prevention of migraine for ages 12–17 years based on a dose of 100 mg daily. Common side effects include cognitive slowing, anorexia, drowsiness, and paresthesias. Blood monitoring should be done for metabolic acidosis. Sodium valproate has been reported to have success in open-label trials of children aged 7–16 years, but a randomized, double-blind, placebo-controlled trial of the extended-release formulation in 300 adolescents aged 12–17 years failed to demonstrate superiority. Commonly reported side effects include weight gain, nausea and abdominal pain, and drowsiness. It has been linked to polycystic ovarian syndrome. Blood monitoring for thrombocytopenia, lymphopenia, and elevations of liver and pancreatic enzymes must be done periodically. Both agents are teratogenic, so birth control measures must be used in females of childbearing age.

The CHAMP study—a multicenter, double-blind, placebo-controlled trial of amitriptyline, topiramate, and placebo in patients aged 18 years or younger with episodic or chronic migraine—was discontinued prematurely because the active arms did not demonstrate superiority over placebo.

OnabotulinumtoxinA has not been formally studied in adolescent migraine patients. Case series and retrospective analyses in teens suggest efficacy at doses of 100–150 units. Similarly, unilateral or bilateral occipital nerve blocks using 2% lidocaine are frequently used in this population of patients with chronic migraine.

Four neuromodulation devices are FDA approved for the treatment of migraine in children and adolescents. For children age 12 and older a noninvasive vagal nerve stimulator (gammaCore) and a noninvasive single-pulse transcranial magnetic stimulator (sTMS mini) are approved for both acute and preventive treatment of migraine, and a remote electrical neuromodulation device (Nerivio) is approved for the treatment of acute attacks. An external trigeminal nerve stimulator (Cefaly) is approved for the acute and prevention treatment of migraine in patients 18 years and older.

The recent practice guideline updates from the American Academy of Neurology and the American Headache Society suggest discussing the various medication options with the patient and families because the active response rates in clinical trials often fail to separate from placebo, the evidence for and adverse effects of amitriptyline plus CBT, topiramate and propranolol, the potential teratogenic consequences of valproate and topiramate, and the need for effective birth control methods and use of folate supplementation when the anticonvulsant medications are prescribed in female adolescents.

Recently, monoclonal antibodies to the calcitonin gene-related peptide (CGRP) ligand or its receptor were approved for the treatment of migraine in adults. Because there is clearly an unmet need for preventive agents in adolescent migraine, and no studies have yet been completed for this age group, the Pediatric and Adolescent Headache Special Interest Group of the American Headache Society published recommendations for their use. These include that these agents be considered primarily for post-pubertal adolescents experiencing eight or more headache days per month, with moderate to severe disability; and that patients should have had adequate trials of, or contraindications to, established migraine prevention, including CBT, neuromodulation devices, and supplements.

Our patient has chronic migraine and has failed treatment with or had contraindications to multiple preventive agents and supplements. She is currently using appropriate nonpharmacologic therapies (CBT and biofeedback) and has no evidence of acute medication overuse. She has never been prescribed a neuromodulation device, and that might be a reasonable next step balancing efficacy and side effect profiles. If therapeutic benefit is not obtained via this method, then a discussion of the benefits and risks of treatment with onabotulinumtoxinA and/or the CGRP monoclonal antibody class should be undertaken with the patient and her family, with emphasis on the fact that neither are FDA approved in adolescents and may not be covered by insurance.

- Migraine affects approximately 20% of adolescents, and chronic migraine affects nearly 2%.
- Chronic migraine has a significant impact on self-esteem, quality of life, social functioning, and scholastic success.
- Preventive should encompass lifestyle modifications and nonpharmacologic and pharmacologic therapies.
- In clinical trials, the active response rates often fail to separate from placebo.
- Only topiramate and 4 neuromodulation devices are FDA approved in this age group.
- The American Headache Society published recommendations for prevention in adolescents.

Further Reading

Green A, Kabbouche M, Kacperski J, Hershet A, O'Brien H. Managing migraine headaches in children and adolescents. *Expert Rev Clin Pharmacol.* 2016;9:477–482.

Hershey AD, Powers SW, Coffey CS, et al. Childhood and Adolescent Migraine Prevention (CHAMP) study: A double-blinded, placebo-controlled, comparative effectiveness study of amitriptyline, topiramate, and placebo in the prevention of childhood and adolescent migraine. *Headache.* 2013;53:799–816.

Hickman C, Lewis KS, Little R, Rastogi RG, Yonker M. Prevention for pediatric and adolescent migraine. *Headache.* 2015;55:1371–1378.

Oskoui M, Pringsheim T, Billinghurst L, et al. Practice guideline update summary: Pharmacologic treatment for pediatric migraine prevention: Report of the Guideline Development, Dissemination, and Implementation Subcommittee of the American Academy of Neurology and the American Headache Society. *Neurology.* 2019;93:500–509.

Papetti L, Ursitti F, Moavero R, et al. Prophylactic treatment of pediatric migraine: Is there anything new in the last decade? *Front Neurol.* 2019;10:771–786.

Szperka C, Vander Pluym J, Orr SL, et al. Recommendations on the use of anti-CGRP monoclonal antibodies in children and adolescents. *Headache.* 2018;58:1658–1669.

Prognostic, Social, and Legal Issues

34 Post-Traumatic Headache

Specialties: Neurology, Primary Care, and Medical Ethics

A 38-year-old man describes severe global headaches since a motor vehicle accident 6 months ago. He does not remember whether or not he struck his head, and he thinks that he did not lose consciousness. He did not seek medical help immediately. Neck pain began the day after the accident, and he recalls that headaches gradually started approximately 1 week to 10 days later. Whereas the neck pain resolved in several days, the headaches have persisted and have been daily. He describes the headaches as throbbing, moderately severe, with nausea, light and sound sensitivity, as well as accompanied by fatigue and malaise. The patient also complains of poor concentration and intermittent dizziness since the accident. He has a prior history of infrequent episodic migraine and depression, but both were under good control before the accident. The headaches and other symptoms have led to the loss of his job (one that he very much valued), and he has been experiencing worsening depression and feelings of hopelessness. The other vehicle in the accident was found to be "at fault." Cervical spine magnetic resonance imaging (MRI) reveals "straightening" and mild midcervical arthritic changes. An MRI of his brain was normal. There is an ongoing lawsuit claiming that permanent damage was done and asking for a multimillion-dollar payment. He wants you to diagnose traumatic causation and to testify to this effect.

What do you do now?

There are threshold legal and career-related questions you must answer first before considering granting your patient's request. You must preliminarily recognize that the word "causation" is a legal term of art that is frequently the subject of hotly contested, expensive litigation in the courts. Be cognizant that assessing causation may also exceed the scope of your duties as a physician in furthering the interests of your patient.

Whether or not a particular event was the causal link for an injury or medical condition suffered by a patient may only be tangentially relevant to your treatment plan, but it is usually not an important factor. Importantly, the exact *opposite* is true for the lawyers handling the case for either the plaintiff or the defendant, and therefore for the patient as well. Thousands of dollars—or even millions—may be at stake based on a medical professional's answer to the question of causation. Consequently, before proceeding to answer it, you should first be fully aware of the legal implications of doing so. If you are employed by an institution or a private practice, you should be equally aware of your employer's policies that may govern your ability to offer such testimony, as well as your employer's view on the financial aspects of your role in the litigation.

Assuming your employer approves or is indifferent to your involvement in litigation, there are legal considerations to think about. First, because providing an opinion on causation normally exceeds the scope of your medical treatment of a patient, you will not receive compensation for the work necessary to provide that opinion from the patient's health insurer or even from the patient directly. Instead, you must first negotiate an agreement with the patient's lawyer or law firm, commonly referred to as a "retainer agreement" or "expert witness agreement." The patient's law firm will normally draft this for you, but it is important to communicate any specific financial terms, such as your hourly rate for expert services, such that they are incorporated into the document before you sign it. It may be advisable to consult with your own lawyer to gain a general understanding of such agreements, if your intention is to provide expert testimony frequently.

Second, be aware that it is highly likely that your opinion on causation will be scrutinized and challenged through a counter-opinion and by cross-examining lawyers. If your patient is the plaintiff in litigation, the defendant's lawyers will be entitled to receive your written report summarizing your findings in advance, after which they can subject you to a deposition at which you will be required to answer questions under oath. A deposition is not the equivalent of a trial; rather, it is a pretrial legal proceeding that allows the opposing lawyers to question you so that they can prepare for a trial that is ordinarily scheduled for many months in the future. At the deposition, lawyers may not question you as aggressively as they would in a case in which causation is not contested. Conversely, if it is contested, you can expect a cross-examination seeking to challenge your causation opinion on any possible ground. Then, if the case proceeds to a trial, you will likely face those lawyers again in front of a jury or judge. In addition, the opposing lawyers may retain their own expert witness, who is frequently a physician in the same area of specialty as you. That expert may also scrutinize your opinion and offer a counter-opinion disagreeing with your opinion. Your patient's lawyers, in turn, may request your time and resources for the purpose of addressing the opposing expert's counter-opinion and for the purpose of preparing for depositions or trials.

Third, you must keep in mind that the U.S. system of justice also offers lawyers, who are considered officers of the court, the option of compelling you to testify whether or not you wish to do so. Lawyers can compel you to testify in most U.S. jurisdictions through a subpoena. However, there are limits on what a subpoena or court order can require you to testify. A court can require you to testify about (1) your observations of the patient based on your memory and (2) the notes you have entered into any medical record. However, a court will not ordinarily require you to testify about causation because the concept of causation exceeds the scope of the treatment you provided to the patient in the past. In effect, requiring you to provide such testimony would be requiring you to provide expert testimony without compensation, which is not the custom and practice of either the legal or the medical profession. Understanding this distinction between testimony regarding past treatment, on the one hand, and testimony about causation, on the other hand, may require you to consult with your own lawyer to ensure that you do not unintentionally trigger legal complications. Violating a court order can lead to serious trouble, and the risk of doing so should always be avoided.

It is only if you are comfortable with the litigation factors described previously that you should agree to provide causation testimony, keeping in mind that testimony about past treatment may be compelled from you regardless of your decision.

If you decide to proceed with providing testimony about causation, the best next steps are to put the legal considerations aside for a moment and first focus on the medical aspects. Start by formulating the proper diagnosis or diagnoses, decide on therapeutic goals with the patient, and think about the best routes for reaching these goals. Putting the legal considerations into a separate category seems to work best because the type of thinking and documentation can be very different from medical models.

In this case, a post-traumatic syndrome seems likely, unless the patient is malingering. Although the latter is possible, it seems unlikely given the highly negative impact his illness has had on his life (no guarantee, of course). The *International Classification of Headache Disorders*, third edition (ICHD-3), defines both headaches attributed to traumatic injury to the head and headache attributed to whiplash (Boxes 34.1 and 34.2), which can become persistent if lasting longer than 3 months, as in this case. There are no specific headache characteristics that define a post-traumatic headache, and the pain often resembles that of either migraine or tension-type headache. However, both diagnoses rest on the appearance of headaches

---

BOX 34.1 **ICHD-3 Acute Headache Attributed to Traumatic Injury to the Head**

DIAGNOSTIC CRITERIA

A. Any headache fulfilling criteria C and D
B. Traumatic injury to the head has occurred.
C. Headache develops within 7 days after one of the following:
   1. The injury to the head
   2. Regaining consciousness after the injury to the head
   3. Discontinuation of medication(s) impairing ability to sense or report headache following the injury to the head
D. Either of the following:
   1. Headache has resolved within 3 months after its onset.
   2. Headache has not yet resolved but 3 months have not yet passed since its onset.
E. Not better accounted for by another ICHD-3 diagnosis

Note: If the headache continues for longer than 3 months, it is coded as persistent headache attributed to traumatic injury to the head.

ICHD-3, *International Classification of Headache Disorders*, third edition.

within 7 days following the injury, and it is not clear whether that time definition holds true in this case. Although there may be many factors involved in the development of these post-traumatic headaches, including axonal injury, neuroinflammation, changes in cerebral metabolism, and genetic predisposition toward developing headache, there is really no clear understanding of how head and neck trauma causes persistent headaches. Analgesic overuse, sleep disturbances, and mood symptoms are all thought to potentially play a role in chronification. Likewise, there are no tests to determine whether an actual injury was done in most cases. Nonetheless, there is significant clinical support for the existence of post-traumatic headaches, sometimes lasting for years, following head trauma (even mild, as in this case) or "whiplash" injury.

This patient's other symptoms—fatigue, malaise during the headaches, and poor concentration and intermittent dizziness at other times—seem to imply a postconcussion syndrome (PCS), defined by the *Diagnostic and Statistical Manual of Mental Disorders*, fourth edition (DSM-IV), as "postconcussional disorder." This controversial disorder can be characterized by the presence of several different symptoms (Box 34.3), the most common of which is headache. Because it is important to use proper terminology, it is worth noting that when the DSM was revised into the fifth edition, the diagnosis of PCS was removed and replaced with "major or mild neurocognitive disorder due to traumatic brain injury," with the

> BOX 34.3   **Symptoms of the Postconcussive Syndrome**
>
> Headaches
> Dizziness, lightheadedness, vertigo
> Visual blurring
> Hearing loss and/or tinnitus
> Fatigue
> Irritability, mood disturbance, anxiety
> Memory, concentration, or other cognitive impairment
> Sleep dysfunction
> Sexual dysfunction

severity label depending on the degree of cognitive symptoms and functional impairment present. The pathophysiology of this condition also remains unknown, although diffuse axonal injury due to acceleration/deceleration forces has been postulated, with most severe effects thought to be present frontotemporally, based on known results of head trauma and autopsy studies.

Many patients with chronic post-traumatic headaches are given psychological diagnoses or are labeled as drug-seeking or malingerers. However, the commonly held belief that a large money settlement will "cure" the syndrome has been shown to be spurious (Packard, 1992). Supporting this patient's legal claim will still be challenging. First, there is likely to be no evidence for brain injury. An MRI of the head can sometimes reveal areas of encephalomalacia or leukomalacia consistent with traumatic brain contusion or other damage sustained at the time of injury, but this is variable. Neuropsychiatric testing can be supportive as well, particularly if the cognitive profile is consistent and the malingering scores are low. A delay in the late cerebral evoked potential P300 can be supportive as well, but this is controversial. Electroencephalography is generally unhelpful unless a seizure focus is found, but functional central nervous system imaging has the potential in the future to be of help. In fact, positron emission tomographic scan abnormalities have been used in legal arguments regarding post-traumatic syndromes.

Another tricky issue is the timing of headache onset because the pain needs to start within 1 week of the injury to meet ICHD-3 criteria, and clinically this may not always be the case. Although this 7-day cutoff may seem arbitrary, the idea of delayed-onset headache is being researched and is mentioned in the Appendix of the ICHD-3. Not an obstacle to the appropriate clinical impression, but one could imagine the opposing attorney brandishing a copy of the ICHD-3 and asking whether or not it is the accepted source for defining headache conditions. On clinical grounds, however, a physician confidently stating a diagnosis can be very compelling. Whether or not to embark on this path is up to the individual physician, but it is important to remember that you might be your patient's only advocate in this situation. All of this obviously requires building trust with your patient. In your note, to promote clarity, it is best to be decisive in documenting your clinical impressions. The legal world tends to disregard the common medical approach of "possible" or "rule-out" diagnoses. So, a reasonable statement in a medical note impression on this case might be "This patient has a post-traumatic headache disorder, more likely than not due to the motor vehicle accident described above." To avoid unmanageable time commitments, many of us find it useful to be available (for a reasonable fee and at specific times) to provide testimony at a deposition but not to make court appearances. Courts generally will recognize and appreciate the time constraints of physicians.

Regarding treatment, despite the lack of good evidence for pharmacological and nonpharmacological options, many patients have been helped by a combination of lifestyle, cognitive–behavioral, and pharmacological therapies. A good place to begin is to perform a thorough search for treatable causes of pain that can be associated with post-traumatic headache, such as occipital or supraorbital neuritis, cervical spine pathology, or other types of musculoskeletal dysfunction, or even other issues such as persistent cerebrospinal fluid leak, traumatic vascular malformations, or cerebral venous thrombosis. Post-traumatic headaches can have many different phenotypes, including ones resembling migraine, tension-type headache, and even cluster headache. What seems to work best in terms of medication choices are those agents with the highest evidence for the specific primary headache phenotype that the post-traumatic headache best resembles, both prophylactically and for the acute relief of breakthrough severe pain.

Here, because this patient's headache is suggestive of a chronic migraine phenotype, a migraine preventive option such as a tricyclic antidepressant or an antiseizure medication might be effective along with lifestyle changes and other approaches discussed in previous chapters. Nonsteroidal anti-inflammatory drugs or possibly even a triptan could be used acutely. Given that he also endorses depression, he should also be referred to see a psychiatrist to better evaluate those symptoms. You as the treating clinician should work closely with his psychiatrist because he will likely do best with this team approach to care.

KEY POINTS TO REMEMBER

- Be aware of threshold legal and career-related questions that must first be answered before you decide whether or not to provide testimony in regard to causation. If you choose to proceed, understand that medical and legal perspectives have different considerations, and there can be differences in what is considered appropriate documentation.
- Mild head and/or neck trauma can lead to chronic headaches, although the specific mechanisms are not clear.
- Headache is commonly a component of PCS.
- Associated injuries to superficial nerves and the cervical spine can be the cause of post-traumatic headaches.
- The ICHD-3 definition of post-traumatic headache requires the onset of head pain within 1 week of the injury, but there are exceptions in clinical practice.

Further Reading

American Psychiatric Association. *Diagnostic and Statistical Manual of Mental Disorders* 4th ed., text rev. Washington, DC: American Psychiatric Association; 2000.

American Psychiatric Association. *Diagnostic and Statistical Manual of Mental Disorders.* 5th ed. Arlington, VA: American Psychiatric Publishing; 2013.

Evans RW. Persistent post-traumatic headache, postconcussion syndrome, and whiplash injuries: The evidence for a non-traumatic basis with an historical review. *Headache.* 2010;50(4):716–724.

Mayer AR, Quinn DK, Master CL. The spectrum of mild traumatic brain injury: A review. *Neurology.* 2017;89(6):623–632.

Pachman S, Lamba A. Legal aspects of concussion: The ever-evolving standard of care. *J Athl Train.* 2017;52(3):186–194.

Packard RC. Posttraumatic headache permanency and relationship to legal settlement. *Headache.* 1992;32:496–500.

35 Headache in the Elderly

Specialties: Neurology and Primary Care

A 75-year-old woman with a prior history of migraine presents for evaluation of frequent headaches.

She states that when she was younger, she would successfully treat acute attacks with sumatriptan but that these headaches have been quiescent for the past 15 years. For the past 6 months, her headaches have returned and occur approximately once or twice per week. She has no other medical illnesses other than mild hypercholesterolemia [total cholesterol 230 mg/dL, high-density lipoprotein (HDL) 70 mg/dL] that is well controlled with simvastatin. She requests a refill of sumatriptan.

What do you do now?

In the United States, people older than age 65 years comprise the fastest growing segment of the population. Migraine is typically thought of as a disease of young people, and although it is true that migraine rarely has its onset after age 50 years and that many individuals with migraine report that their headaches improve as they grow older, the prevalence of migraine in the elderly is significant. Estimates suggest that 3–10% of those older than age 65 years suffer from migraine, report migraine-related disability, and require treatment.

It is also very important to note that this patient is experiencing new headache after a remission of migraine for several years. The first task is to ensure this is indeed a migraine recurrence and not a secondary headache. We can accomplish this by taking a careful history and performing a detailed exam, as well as requesting imaging, blood work, and other tests as appropriate. In this age group, secondary headaches, such as giant cell arteritis, cervicogenic headache, occipital neuralgia, cardiac cephalalgia, hypnic headache, and headache secondary to subacute glaucoma, become more of a risk and need to be screened for when a patient presents with new headache.

Provided that we have done a thorough workup for secondary causes, and none have been found, we are left with the diagnosis of migraine. The use of triptans in the elderly raises several important clinical issues. Some clinicians have an arbitrary age limit above which they do not prescribe these medications; others will use these agents as long as there are no medical contraindications. Given that these agents were not tested in the elderly, the increased risk of medical comorbidities (especially cardiac and cerebrovascular diseases) and polypharmacy that occurs in older patients, as well as the changes in drug metabolism and elimination that may occur as patients age, the decision-making process here is difficult. Many patients who began using these medications decades ago have now reached the age at which their health care providers are uncomfortable with or unwilling to continue prescribing. In the absence of formal guidelines, how do we decide?

The package inserts for all the triptans state that these medications are contraindicated for patients with risk factors for coronary artery disease (CAD) unless they have undergone a "thorough cardiovascular evaluation" that provides "satisfactory clinical evidence" that cardiovascular disease has been excluded. These package inserts do not specify what this evaluation should include. Some clinicians interpret this to mean that all patients who are at risk for cardiac disease be screened with electrocardiography (ECG) and stress tests prior to being prescribed triptans. Yet, the limitations of these tests to document asymptomatic CAD are well described, and in fact those same package inserts state "the sensitivity of cardiac diagnostic procedures to detect cardiovascular disease or predisposition to coronary artery vasospasm is modest, at best." Because of these limitations, some have proposed that this cardiac evaluation consist of risk factor stratification based on results from the Framingham Study. This model incorporates six variables (gender, total cholesterol levels, HDL levels, blood pressure, presence or absence of diabetes, and tobacco use) and is capable of providing reliable 10-year estimates of a patient's CAD risk. This method allows patients to be stratified into low (<10% risk of symptomatic CAD within the next 10 years), intermediate (>10% but <20%), or high (>20%) risk groups.

Patients often report that their migraine attacks become less severe with advancing age. For these patients, a trial of a previously ineffective symptomatic medication may be warranted. Remember, however, that nonsteroidal anti-inflammatory drugs and aspirin may also be more likely to induce bleeding in the elderly and may interact with other medications frequently also prescribed for these patients. Acetaminophen and other analgesics may be metabolized differently in the elderly and need to be more closely monitored. For patients who continue to experience disabling headaches and in whom risk stratification is low, triptans can be prescribed. Patients with an intermediate level of risk require further cardiac evaluation. If stress testing is normal, then triptans may be prescribed. In any event, the physician should clearly document in the chart that the patient suffers from disabling migraine that has failed to respond to other therapies, that the risks and benefits were discussed with the patient, and that the patient believes that the benefits outweigh the risks. Patients in the high-risk category should not be prescribed triptans.

In addition to her age, this patient's only known risk factors for CAD is mild hypercholesterolemia, which is well controlled with medication. Using a calculator to determine her Framingham risk (http://www.cardiol ogy.org/tools/medcalc/fram), we can determine that her estimate of a cardiovascular event is 1% over 5 years and 4% over 10 years. The patient is therefore in the low-risk category and can use a triptan. She will have documentation placed into her chart that she understands the risks and benefits as discussed previously. She will continue to be followed closely at regular intervals; should new risk factors for cardiovascular or cerebrovascular disease develop or other medical conditions arise, her medication regimen may need to be adjusted.

Unfortunately, there are many individuals who are ineligible for triptan therapy because of their medical comorbidities. Until recently, this group had few choices for acute treatment. However, with the recent U.S. Food and Drug Administration approvals of lasmiditan, a serotonin 1F receptor agonist, which is now the first "ditan" available, and the calcitonin gene-related peptide small-molecule antagonists ubrogepant and rimegepant (referred to as "gepants"), new acute treatments that lack vasoconstriction activity are now available and provide new options.

KEY POINTS TO REMEMBER

- When an older individual presents with new-onset headache, this is a red flag and secondary causes must be excluded.
- There is no evidence that age alone is a contraindication to triptan use.
- Routine screening with ECG and stress testing is costly and not sensitive in patients with asymptomatic CAD.
- For patients without known cardiovascular disease, treatment recommendations should be based on risk stratification from the Framingham Study.
- Low-risk patients can be prescribed triptans.
- High-risk patients should avoid triptans.
- Intermediate-risk patients need more focused cardiac evaluations with ECG and stress testing.

Further Reading

Bravo TP. Headaches of the elderly. *Curr Neurol Neurosci Rep.* 2015;15:30.

Dodick D, Lipton RB, Martin V. Consensus statement: Cardiovascular safety profile of triptans (5-HT1B/1D agonists) in the acute treatment of migraine. *Headache.* 2004;44(5):414.

Krege JH, Rizzoli PB, Liffick E, et al. Safety findings from phase 3 lasmiditan studies for acute treatment of migraine: Results from SAMURAI and SPARTAN. *Cephalalgia.* 2019;39(8):957–966.

Loder E, Biondi D. Can this patient take a triptan? Review of the cardiovascular safety of the triptans and recommendations for patient selection and evaluation. *Internet J Neurol.* 2004;3:1–15.

Prencipe M, Casini AR, Ferretti C, et al. Prevalence of headache in an elderly population: Attack frequency, disability, and use of medication. *J Neurol Neurosurg Psychiatry.* 2001;70(3):377–381.

Ward TN. Headache disorders in the elderly. *Curr Treat Options Neurol.* 2002;4(5):403–408.

Recurring Headaches
in Medication-Averse
Patients

A 28-year-old teacher reports headaches accompanied
by nausea and sensitivity to light, sound, and
movement since his teens but worsening in college.
They occur "several" times each month, although
frequency varies, and they can last all day. They
sometimes disable him from work, and he has missed
several days in the past several months. He is an avid
yoga practitioner and states that it has clearly helped
with headaches. He takes a number of supplements,
including vitamin D, vitamin C, a B vitamin complex,
turmeric, and *S*-adenosine-l-methionine (SAM-e).

What do you do now?

When patients are averse to pharmaceutical intervention, it is worthwhile exploring their reasons, many of which can be quite valid, including previous intolerable adverse effects. Clearly, overaggressive attempts to alter their preferences might be counterproductive, leading to a lack of trust and poor compliance. On the other hand, listening to their specific concerns and addressing them when possible might set the stage for introducing low-risk and well-tolerated medication, perhaps starting with very low dosages, in conjunction with nonpharmaceutical measures. These options are discussed in the following sections and summarized in Table 36.1.

NUTRICEUTICALS

This category generally includes plant-derived treatments—which include oral preparations, topical preparations, and inhaled forms ("aromatherapy")—and "supplements" (usually minerals and vitamins). There are many options in these categories, yet evidence supporting their use is sparse. This is in part due to the wide range of doses and forms available for these agents, as well as the fact that little funding has been available for doing proper investigations.

Butterbur, derived from the root of the plant *Petasites hybridus*, has good evidence for suppressing migraine prophylactically. Unfortunately, it

TABLE 36.1 **Selected Herbal and Other Supplements Useful in Migraine**

Supplement	Derivation	Dose
Riboflavin (vitamin B$_2$)	Synthetic/plant-derived	400 mg daily
Magnesium	Synthetic (e.g., gluconate, glycinate)	600 mg daily
Feverfew	Leaf	50 mg daily
Ginger	Root	Candied lozenges prn
Coenzyme Q10	Synthetic/plant-derived	150–300 mg daily
Boswellia	Resin	400 mg daily

seemed to be hepatotoxic in a few individuals. There is reasonable evidence that some preparations are safe, but uncertainty has discouraged its use. Feverfew has very little supportive evidence and because the portions of the plant that help (leaves) contain salicylates, there could be risks similar to those with aspirin. Melatonin is available from plant sources and is supported by some evidence for migraine prevention (see Table 36.1). Boswellia, made from the resin of the *Boswellia serrata* tree, has some supportive evidence for pain prophylaxis in general and has helped a number of migraine patients, particularly as adjunctive therapy.

Cannabis has long been touted as a headache remedy, but there is virtually no evidence of its benefits acutely or prophylactically. The isolated cannabinoid cannabidiol (CBD) seemed to hold promise, but to date this has not been apparent except in selected cases. Ginger root does seem efficacious for nausea but not particularly active in headache.

Magnesium supplementation does seem to help some patients with migraine in the dose range of 400–600 mg daily. Loose stools limit its use in some. In small studies, riboflavin and coenzyme Q (both involved in the electron transport chain metabolism) have been shown to help prevent migraine at doses of 400 mg daily and 150–300 mg daily, respectively.

Topical therapy does not seem to benefit migraine patients other than its possible "aromatherapy" benefits, with peppermint, eucalyptus, and lavender mentioned most frequently.

BEHAVIORAL TREATMENT

Strong evidence for the effectiveness of some behavioral treatments in migraine suggests that these are underutilized in current medical environments. Relaxation training, with or without physiological measures (biofeedback), can be not only useful but also empowering psychologically for patients who are frustrated by the lack of control they feel over their migraine condition. Moderate regular exercise, tailored to the individual's capacity, is helpful in many cases but sometimes takes a level of commitment that is difficult to achieve. Similarly, avoiding triggering activities such as overusing alcohol and caffeine, overeating, and not practicing good sleep hygiene is extremely important but difficult to ensure.

Cognitive–behavioral therapy has been promoted, but evidence is not clear. Better evidence seems to be emerging for mindfulness meditative training and activity, although more work needs to be done regarding best formats and duration for these.

ELECTRICAL AND MAGNETIC STIMULATION

With the hope of altering neural circuitry responsible for ongoing migraine, electrical neuromodulation techniques have resurfaced recently. Transcutaneous nerve stimulation (TENS) of the supraorbital nerve bundles (Cefaly®) and of the vagus nerve (Gammacore®) have their adherents and have some reasonable evidence to support prophylactic and acute use. Nerivio Migra® is a new stimulation device worn on the upper arm that has some supportive evidence in migraine. Transcranial magnetic stimulation also seems useful, particularly for people with bothersome migraine with aura.

PHYSICAL TECHNIQUES

Massage has clearly been effective for some patients, but it is limited by accessibility and affordability. In addition, it has proven virtually impossible to study in a blinded controlled manner. Acupuncture continues to be unsupported by solid evidence for migraine but has been of use in selected patients. Chiropractic has likewise never been shown to help prevent migraine.

Our patient has migraine attacks at a frequency high enough to warrant both acute and preventive measures. He will appreciate active listening to his concerns, and it will be important to gain his trust if previous clinicians have been less attentive. It is also important, however, to ensure he understands that some supplements are potentially harmful, particularly because they are much less tightly regulated. He is currently taking vitamin D, which is extremely popular and may in fact be useful in some patients with migraine, but it may also build up in the system and become toxic. Similarly, SAM-e has no real evidence for effectiveness and might not be entirely without risk. A good place to start might be to suggest behavioral treatments and aromatherapy with peppermint oil, along with a pharmacological rescue medication with a very tolerable adverse effect profile, such as naratriptan.

- Some herbal and other nonpharmacological treatments are safe and may be very useful. However, it is important for patients to understand that these may be nonbenign and should be scrutinized carefully.
- Some people with migraine and other headaches who are averse to medication will respond to practitioners who listen to their concerns and creatively design treatment programs with their preferences in mind, including perhaps low-dose medications as trials.
- Behavioral treatments have good evidence supporting their use in headache prophylaxis and should always be considered as adjuncts to other therapy.

Further Reading

Irby MB, Bond DS, Lipton RB, Nicklas B, Houle TT, Penzien DB. Aerobic exercise for reducing migraine burden: Mechanisms, markers, and models of change processes. *Headache*. 2016;56:357–369.

Levin M. Herbal treatment of headache. *Headache*. 2012;52:76–80.

Mauskop A. *The Headache Alternative: A Neurologist's Guide to Drug-Free Relief*. New York, NY: Dell; 1997.

Wells RE, Seng EK, Edwards RR, et al. Mindfulness in migraine: A narrative review. *Expert Rev Neurotherapeut*. 2020;20:207–225.

37 COVID-19 Cephalalgia

A 53-year-old man who has been under your care for his migraine without aura calls to arrange an urgent appointment. He tells you that for the past 3 days he has had a global, moderate to severe throbbing headache that does not respond to his typical anti-migraine medications. Today, he awoke with a mild sore throat, body aches, a temperature of 100.2°F, and noticed that his sense of smell was gone. Two weeks ago, he attended a family barbeque at which no one wore masks, but he said no one at the gathering was sick.

What do you do now?

This patient most likely has a viral illness accounting for his symptoms. However, his complaint of anosmia in addition to the low-grade fever, myalgias, sore throat, and new-onset headache suggests that he may have early symptoms of COVID-19.

COVID-19, caused by the severe acute respiratory syndrome coronavirus 2 (SARS-CoV-2), was first reported in patients in Wuhan, China, in December 2019 and declared a pandemic by the World Health Organization in March 2020. Although the disease predominantly presents with respiratory manifestations, the virus also has an affinity for the gastroenterological, hematological, renal, and neurological systems.

Neurologic complications of COVID-19 may be due to direct invasion by the virus, an autoimmune response against the virus, metabolic derangements, hypercoagulability, or other neurological complications resulting from the systemic effects of the virus. The SARS-CoV-2 virus can attack essentially any part of the nervous system. Central nervous system (CNS) manifestations include headache, meningitis, encephalitis, seizures, and stroke.

Headache appears to be a common symptom, affecting up to 75% of patients infected with the novel coronavirus. The exact mechanism by which SARS-CoV-2 produces headache is not yet known. Putative mechanisms include entry into the brain through the olfactory bulb, a similar entry point believed to be used by the herpes simplex virus; direct viral infection across the blood–brain barrier (BBB); or as the result of the cytokine storm that follows SARS-CoV-2 infection.

In mouse models, intranasal injection of the human coronavirus OC43 has been documented to cause CNS spread. This route of viral entry seems plausible given that anosmia and ageusia are seen commonly with COVID-19 infections and can occur as the sole symptoms or with other clinical features. In a multicenter European study, 86% of COVID-19 patients reported anosmia. Using this as a portal of entry, the virus could directly invade trigeminal nerve endings in the nasal cavity, producing an inflammatory cascade to cause headache.

Transport across the BBB following viremia or when carried via infected leukocytes may permit the virus to enter the glia cells and neurons by binding to angiotensin-converting enzyme 2 receptors. These receptors are found in the brain vascular endothelium and smooth muscle. One could speculate that the endothelial cells could trigger activation of the trigeminovascular pathways, leading to head pain.

Although there is no strong evidence that the SARS-Co-2 virus is highly neurovirulent, perhaps the headache and other CNS symptomatology are the result of the immunological response to the virus. Cytokine storm, an overexaggerated immunologic reaction, has been well documented with COVID infection. Increased levels of the proinflammatory cytokines [interleukin (IL)-2, IL-6, IL-7, IL-10, granulocyte colony-stimulating factor, interferon-γ-inducible protein 10, tumor necrosis factor, and others] have been measured in the plasma of infected individuals. These cytokines can cause pain through direct tissue injury and a subsequent inflammatory cascade that potentially could cause headache through activation of the perivascular trigeminal nerve endings.

Several studies have detailed the clinical features of COVID-19 headaches. That headache is a common feature of COVID-19 is not surprising because systemic viral illnesses often cause headaches that are not well characterized (Box 37.1). Bolay et al. (2020) reported that the headaches associated with COVID-19 in their practice in Turkey occurred in approximately 10% of symptomatic patients and were a predominant reason for patients seeking medical care. The headaches were bilateral, pulsating or pressure-like, of moderate to severe intensity, and usually located in the temporoparietal region or forehead, periorbital, or sinus areas. The headaches were sudden or gradual in onset, resistant to analgesics, and associated with photo- and phonophobia. In their report, the headaches were limited to the active phase of the illness. More recently, two studies from Spanish Emergency Departments provided more insights into the COVID-related headaches. In one study, 68% of confirmed or probable cases reported headaches. In the patients with confirmed COVID-19, there was an increased incidence of anosmia. In most cases, the headache appeared simultaneously with the other symptoms. In this series of 145 patients, the headache was most often bilateral (87%), and holocephalic or frontal pain was reported by 34%. The headache was pressure-like in one-third of patients, throbbing in 11%, and associated with photophobia (29%) and phonophobia (27%). Head pain was exacerbated by coughing, physical activity, and fever. In the 25% of patients with pre-existing migraine, nearly all reported that the COVID headache was different than their usual. Caronna et al. (2020) reported that 75% of their patients presenting to the emergency department with COVID reported headache. These patients reported anosmia/ageusia more often than did those without headache. Severe pain with migraine-like features was seen in 25%. Interestingly, they found that headache associated with COVID-19 was predictive of a shorter course of the disease. The authors also reported that one-third of the patients had persistent, disabling headaches unresponsive to acute therapies as the only sequala of the infection, and half of those patients had no prior headache history.

In my practice (LN), I have seen several presentations of headaches associated with COVID infection, depending on the phase of the infection (Table 37.1). Several patients who were presymptomatic complained of new-onset stabbing headaches beginning several days before the onset of fever, cough, and myalgias, resolving as these symptoms emerged. Others

TABLE 37.1 **Possible Causes of COVID-19 Cephalalgia**

Primary	Secondary
Migraine	Viral associated
Tension-type	Headache associated with hypoxia/hypercapnia
Cough	Stroke
Stabbing	Cortical vein thrombosis
Exertional	Sagittal sinus thrombosis
New daily persistent headache	Meningitis
	Encephalitis
	Headache attributed to exposure to other substances, cytokines
	Cough
	Stabbing
	Exertional

developed global, throbbing headaches that accompanied the onset of symptoms and that, like typical viral headaches, worsened with increases in fever. Similar to the patients reported on by Bolay et al. (2020), these patients had no relief with analgesics. In my patients with pre-existing migraine, all described their COVID-19–related headaches as distinct from their typical head pains and unresponsive to triptans or analgesics. Several patients, without a prior history of headache, reported a global, throbbing headache without any associated symptoms beginning during the active infection and persisting unabated for the past 3 months, meeting criteria for new daily persistent headache (see Chapter 7).

Our patient should be instructed to not make an office visit because there is a high likelihood that he has COVID-19. His concerns should be addressed on the telephone or preferably on a telemedicine visit, and he should be instructed to consult with his primary care physician or internist and to get urgent care should his condition worsen. He should also be instructed to self-quarantine and to call the other people with whom he interacted to alert them of his probable infectious status so that they can be tested and isolate.

If his neurological exam is normal, and no other red flags exist, his headache could be treated symptomatically with prescription nonsteroidal anti-inflammatory drugs (NSAIDs) if there are no contraindications (the warning to avoid NSAIDs early in the pandemic has been discounted), although as mentioned previously, these headaches seem to be resistant to analgesics.

If his exam is abnormal, or if nuchal rigidity, alterations in mental status, or neurologic deficits develop, he and his family members must be instructed to seek emergency department care. The clinician should be vigilant because COVID-19 can cause a hypercoagulable state and headache may be a result of a stroke or cortical vein/sagittal sinus thromboses. Similarly, meningitis and encephalitis have been reported with SARS-CoV-2 infections and must be considered in the differential diagnoses for headache in this setting.

KEY POINTS TO REMEMBER

- COVID-19 may cause neurological complications involving any part of the neuroaxis.
- Headaches are reported in as many of 40% of those affected by the SARS-CoV-2 virus and are usually resistant to analgesics.
- COVID-19–related headaches may be caused by activation of the trigeminal–vascular pathways by viral entry into the brain through the olfactory bulb, direct viral infection across the BBB, or as the result of the cytokine storm that follows SARS-CoV-2 infection.
- The headache of COVID-19 may have characteristics that resemble migraine or be nonspecific like other headaches associated with systemic viral infections.
- If abnormalities are found on the neurological exam, a workup for sinister causes of headaches must be undertaken (see Table 37.1).

Further Reading

Berger JR. COVID-19 and the nervous system. *J Neurovirol*. 2020;26:143–148.

Bobker SM, Robbins MS. COVID-19 and headache: A primer for trainees. *Headache*. 2020;60(8):1806–1811.

Bolay H, Gul A, Baykan B. Views and perspectives: COVID-19 is a real headache! Headache 2020;60(7):1415–1421.

Caronna E, Ballve A, Llaurado A, et al. Headache: A striking prodromal and persistent symptom, predictive of COVID-19 clinical evolution. *Cephalalgia*. 2020;40(13):1410–1421.

Ellul MA, Benjamin L, Singh B, et al. Neurological associations of COVID-19. *Lancet Neurol*. 2020;19(9):767–783.

MaasenVanDenBrink A, de Vries T, Danser AHJ. Headache medication and the COVID-19 pandemic. *J Headache Pain*. 2020;21(1):38.

Membrilla JA, de Lorenzo I, Sastre M, Diaz deTeran J. Headache as a cardinal symptom of coronavirus disease 2019: A cross-sectional study. *Headache*. 2020;60(10):2176–2191.

Index

Tables, figures, and boxes are indicated by *t*, *f*, and *b* following the page number

migraine (*cont.*)
    preventive therapy, in children, 174
    side-locked, differential diagnosis, 68
    sporadic hemiplegic, 48
    TNF-α levels, 39
    treatment, 12, 86, 103, 114, 116–17
    treatment success/refractoriness, 102–3
    vestibular (*see* vestibular migraine)
    without aura, diagnostic criteria, 11*b*
    WMH differential diagnosis, 16–18,
        16f
migraine/aura
    characterization, 48–50, 48*b*, 52
    diagnostic criteria, 49*b*
    imaging, 50–51
    migraine aura status, 50
    motor auras, 52
    oral contraceptives, 152–55, 163–66
    pregnancy-associated, 157–62
    stroke risk, 153, 155, 165
    subclasses, 50, 52
    suicidal ideation, 142–44
    treatment, 51, 51*b*
migraine/chronic
    addiction-associated, 145–47
    in adolescents, 175, 179–83
    characterization, 130
    diagnostic criteria, 130*b*
    diagnostic workup, 112, 116
    differential diagnosis, 112, 113
    HIV-associated, 115–17
    nerve blocks, 132, 133
    preventive therapy, 130–33, 131*b*,
        180–81
    refractory, 129–33
    treatment, 112–14, 113*b*, 116–17
    wearing-off phenomenon, 131–33
migraine with brainstem aura
    characterization, 54
    diagnostic criteria, 55*b*
    differential diagnosis, 55, 57*t*, 58
migrainous infarction, 50, 52
mood disorders, 141–44

multiple sclerosis
    brainstem plaque, differential diagnosis, 57*t*
    Dawson's fingers, 17
    evaluation of, 18
    management, 18–19
    WMH, differential diagnosis, 17–18
muscle relaxants, 109

naproxen
    childhood migraine, 174
    cough headache, 65
    menstrual migraine, 152, 154*t*
    pregnancy-associated migraine, 159–60
naratriptan, 154*t*, 174–75, 176*t*, 204
nasal septal deviation, 12
NDPH. *see* new daily persistent headache
neoplasms
    acoustic nerve region tumors, 55
    brain, 5
    brainstem tumor, 57*t*
    differential diagnosis, 64
    intracranial mass, 68
    scalp infection/mass, 68, 108
Nerivio, 181–82, 204
nerve blocks
    cranial, 92
    migraine/chronic, 132, 133
    occipital, 40, 132, 161, 181
    sphenopalatine, 132
neuromodulation
    adolescent migraine, 181–82
    childhood migraine, 176
    NDPH, 40
Neurontin. *see* gabapentin
neurostimulation, 161
new daily persistent headache
    characterization, 38
    diagnostic criteria, 38*b*
    differential diagnosis, 38
    etiology, 39
    evaluation of, 38–39
    pain-reducing techniques, 40
    treatment, 39–40